Ineke Meredith was born in New Zealand to parents of mixed-Samoan heritage. She spent part of her childhood in Samoa but moved to New Zealand to study medicine.

She is a general surgeon with a subspecialty interest in breast cancer and breast reconstruction who has published research articles in international peer-reviewed medical journals on breast cancer and reconstruction, cancer rates among Pacific peoples in New Zealand, and has participated in international collaboratives on cancer rates in diaspora. She is the founder and director of Fur Love, a canine skincare company, and lives and works between New Zealand and Paris.

T0323266

On
Call

INEKE MEREDITH

On Call

HarperCollins*Publishers*

CONTENT WARNING
On Call contains descriptions of medical procedures that may be confronting or disturbing for some readers, as well as references to end-of-life care and death.

HarperCollins*Publishers*
Australia • Brazil • Canada • France • Germany • Holland • India
Italy • Japan • Mexico • New Zealand • Poland • Spain • Sweden
Switzerland • United Kingdom • United States of America

First published in 2024
by HarperCollins*Publishers* (New Zealand) Limited
Unit D1, 63 Apollo Drive, Rosedale, Auckland 0632, New Zealand
harpercollins.co.nz

Copyright © Ineke Meredith 2024

Ineke Meredith asserts the moral right to be identified as the author of this work. This work is copyright. All rights reserved. No part of this publication may be reproduced, copied, scanned, stored in a retrieval system, recorded, or transmitted, in any form or by any means, without the prior written permission of the publisher. Without limiting the author's and publisher's exclusive rights, any unauthorized use of this publication to train generative artificial intelligence (AI) technologies is expressly prohibited.

A catalogue record for this book is available from the National Library of New Zealand

ISBN 978 1 7755 4237 7 (pbk)
ISBN 978 1 7754 9268 9 (ebook)

Cover design by Louisa Maggio, HarperCollins Design Studio
Cover photography by Rachel Calvo
Typeset in Bembo Std by Kirby Jones
Printed and bound in the UK using 100% Renewable Electricity at CPI Group (UK) Ltd

Dedicated to the patients I have had the immense privilege of treating, to my registrars, who inspire me, and to my son, husband, family and friends, who love me no matter what

CONTENTS

Prologue

I hate the phone. Especially when it rings in the middle of the night. It had barely rung once by the time I answered it, but to sleep while on call is to sleep awake, if that exists. Paranoia over missing a call prevails over fatigue, and years of practice have trained my ears so well I jumped on that call before the second ring could start. It was 2 a.m., and the voice on the other end told me there had been a car accident. 'This is a trauma call. There has been a major road traffic accident. Multiple victims. ETA ten minutes.'

In the lonely darkness of my hotel room, I pulled on jeans and sneakers, then drove the even lonelier streets to the hospital. I was filled with regret. Not because I didn't love my job and what I did, but because I hated the loneliness. The loneliness of a phone ringing in the dark to announce an emergency. The loneliness of getting into the car when everyone else is already dreaming of tomorrow. The loneliness of a hospital at night – it is cold and empty and sound reverberates off the stark white walls in a way it doesn't in daylight. And, as was the case on this particular night, the loneliness of standing in the emergency department before two mangled 15-year-old bodies.

On my two-minute drive to the hospital, the eerily empty streets had given no hint of the police chase that had taken place when a trio of teenage boys stole a car from the next town over. There had been no evidence of the driver losing control of the vehicle, no evidence of the car smashing into a lamp post at high speed and being torn in half. One of the boys had apparently survived the impact and run away from the scene. His friends had not been so fortunate.

Both boys were motionless, lying in adjacent resuscitation rooms on hospital trolleys. In a larger hospital, these rooms would have been filled with staff – emergency, anaesthetics, intensive care, surgery, nursing staff, orderlies, machines, drugs, equipment – but these boys, critical from the moment they'd been extricated from the vehicle, did not have such an audience. In small hospitals, staffing is minimal. There was one anaesthetist and one surgeon (me), along with two junior doctors. The two small resuscitation rooms were strangely empty. Where was everyone else?

The first boy was bleeding profusely out of his ears and nose. When I put my hand against him, he was warm. Then I looked at the heart-rate monitor and felt anxiety mounting in the back of my throat. He was unstable – his heart was beating rapidly, his blood pressure was dangerously low, and he was behaving like he had lost a large volume of blood. 'Floor and four more,' I whispered to myself. Chest, abdomen, pelvis, long bones, floor: these are the places people can hide internal blood loss. It had been drummed into us through training. Floor and four more; if you can't find it in the four, never forget to check the floor.

I already knew the blood coming out of his ears and nose was not a problem I could fix. It meant a serious head injury, but confirming that would have required a CT scan of his head, and that was impossible until he was stable enough to lie in the scanner. A bedside ultrasound showed fluid in his abdomen, and I hoped that meant there would be bleeding I *could* control. Blood replacement and fluids were administered, but he descended quickly into cardiac arrest, and cardiopulmonary resuscitation was commenced.

'Let's go to theatre,' I said once he was shocked back into a rhythm, hoping I might be able to control any bleeding inside his abdomen or pelvis, then get him transferred to the tertiary centre 150 kilometres away. My own heart was pounding, my ears ringing, the high-pitched and urgent beeping of the cardiac monitors bouncing off the walls of the empty corridors. Then, as the anaesthetist and I wheeled the boy to the operating block, I saw the junior doctors commencing CPR on the other boy, and with each chest compression my own distress grew.

Shit, I thought. I can't do this alone. Maybe I do hate this job.

* * *

'It's so quiet here,' I had been told when I'd taken the locum weekend as the surgeon on call. 'Nothing ever happens.'

The town was quaint, full of vineyards and restaurants, and my first day had been uneventful. After attending the morning round with the team, I'd gone for a long lunch with a friend. Later on, at 10 p.m., I'd been informed that there were no potential surgical patients in the emergency department, and that there had been no referrals from the community. This was good news, and I'd nurtured some hope of a full night's sleep. Of course, I should have known better.

After calling for an intensive care doctor to be helicoptered urgently from the tertiary hospital, I had taken that first boy to theatre and made a big incision into his abdominal cavity. He had a small haematoma behind his colon, but that was not the cause of his rapid heart rate and low blood pressure. The remainder of his abdomen was pristine. I could not see a reason for the instability. By this point, his blood was no longer clotting and he was bleeding profusely from everywhere he could. This is a very bad sign. *Pre-mortem*. He died on the table.

Before I had finished closing him up, I felt a tap on my shoulder. It was the intensive care doctor, who upon arrival had thrown himself into resuscitating the second boy. 'You

4

need to bring him to theatre too,' he said. It was a copy-paste situation. The boy clearly had a major head injury, and yet I had to inflict another wound from the bottom of his ribcage to the top of his pubic bone, where we looked for bleeding in his abdominal cavity. But again there was very little intra-abdominal bleeding to account for his degree of instability. Again we were looking for an alternative reason for his circulatory failure. Again he arrested on the table.

By the end of the night, both of the boys were dead.

It was daylight by the time I exited the hospital. There were police cars outside and I did not make eye contact. Back in my hotel room, I stood underneath a scalding-hot shower, my whole body in pain. My legs ached, my neck was constantly in spasm and my shoulders were so sore I could not wear a bra. I wondered whether 'battle fatigue' was a term used exclusively for soldiers. I was wrung out, and I felt guilty for the comfort that the hot water and then the clean sheets on my bed gave me. Lying there, I replayed the night's events, my ears ringing, my thoughts flying as I questioned what I could have done differently for those boys. I was afraid to close my eyes for what I might see behind them. But I also knew I had to sleep. I had a full list the next day.

* * *

I first knew I wanted to do general surgery when, as a junior doctor, I saw an emergency transfer of a young woman who had sustained major trauma to the blood vessels in her pelvis. When the helicopter arrived, I had watched as she was carried out on a trolley, intubated and ventilated, with a general surgeon sitting on top of her. She had been transferred with her lower abdomen open and his fist deep in her pelvis, pushed firmly against the fatal injury in order to stem the bleeding and get her to more advanced care. His fist had saved her life.

When I saw that, I wanted it. Then I lived it. I thrived on it, and I loved it. But the day after losing those two boys, I just felt a wreck. There is no down-time in surgery. Even less when you try to keep the rest of your life afloat. I had reached my end.

In fact, I had been toying with that end for a while. I had seen my colleagues give up their lives for the profession, operate through the night, cancel family plans, receive angry phone calls – from spouses, from patients, from secretaries, from nurses – for being late, as if they might have been having coffee somewhere in the sun and not in theatre, operating in emergencies. Let's be honest, they would have rather been somewhere else. Then I had seen these same colleagues leave, exhausted, their contributions to the hospital briefly acknowledged in token afternoon teas.

Everyone I knew was angry or worn out, and as I had stood there in the shower – unable to think, worried about the pain in my neck and the big caseload I had scheduled for the next day, unable to gather enough energy to be better for those I loved – I knew I could not be in that same position in another year. I simply would not allow that to happen. I was already full of regret for what I had not given my mother. Something had to change.

* * *

Of course, I loved surgery. The messiness, the intensity, the strange people who choose it as a career. And, despite the drama, some of my most memorable moments as a surgeon are not, in fact, the horrific traumas or the lengthy middle-of-the-night theatre escapades. There are also the moments of softness. The heartbreaking acknowledgements that life will no longer be the same after first cancer diagnoses, the tears between fathers and sons, mothers and daughters when a cancer has recurred, the silent goodbyes between husbands and wives.

This book is an illustration of my path as a general surgeon. The madness of a day's work. The cases that, by touching me a little too closely, broke my heart and enlightened me in equal parts. It's a story of the good, the bad and the crazy. And it's also a testament to the bravery of a doctor's patients and what they can endure.

But, as you read it, please remember that I am actually a very happy person. I just do not think I was prepared.

1.

Chaos and the dancing star

For my eighth birthday, I wanted a ruler. A roller ruler, with which I could draw not only straight lines but circles too. However, at $15 a pop, it was a little ostentatious, so I had to stick with my ordinary ruler, which was limited to straight lines.

To save money, and because she was creative, my mother taught herself to sew and, much to my embarrassment, I had to wear home-made clothes to school. It was the late 1980s, and my mother's preoccupation with Whitney Houston meant I ended up with a horribly distinctive red leopard-print dress with bulky shoulder pads. As if I did not already have enough to deal with. I was already teased for looking 'different', thanks to my fuller lips, the dark hair on my forearms and the fact that my father was my hairdresser. The other kids were fair-skinned, blond-haired, had 'normal'-sized lips, and I am pretty sure their fathers did not cut their hair.

I was born in New Zealand, where I spent the first eight years of my life, before my parents moved me and my three siblings back to their home country, Samoa, an island in the South Pacific. There, we all lived in one room, the six of us sharing two beds for two years. When the fifth child arrived, we moved into a three-bedroom home. Moving to Samoa was somewhat of a culture shock. The students at school called me 'white', so it seemed that I just could not fit in with a group of my peers at that age. At my new school, which was Catholic, I quickly learnt two important things: the rosary, and that if you could not recite it to perfection the nuns would strike you. After the second time I received a thump on the back, I refused to go back to that horrible place, where all the students looked at me as if I was an alien. I was moved to the main public school in the capital.

My father was a religious man, but he was particularly zealous on Sundays. That is, he went to work during the week, did not speak kindly to his wife, did not share knowledge with his children, liked to drink alcohol on Friday and Saturday nights with his friends, beat his wife and children when he did not get the answers he was looking for, and without fail went to church every Sunday. Not only that, but he would drag his entire family (who he had just spent the entire morning screaming at) to sit in the front pew, as close as possible to Jesus on the crucifix. Somehow, despite his religious emancipation, he was particularly intolerable on Sundays.

I would feel my father's wrath for laughing, or for boys calling the house. Unfortunately for me, my neighbour did not know that. He did not know that his every unwelcome attempt at contact fuelled my father's fire. I was 14 years old, not far from turning 15, when my neighbourhood admirer, spurred on by peripubertal testosterone, came to the door uninvited, wrote my name in spray paint all over the lamp posts around our house, and called our landline after 7 p.m. – a time when *no one* was allowed to call and the mere sound of the phone would fill us all with dread. One evening a 7.15 p.m. call came, and I meekly and hastily told my neighbour I couldn't talk while my father stood curling his lips in anger.

'Who was that?' he said menacingly when I hung up.

'I don't know!' I yelled back in exasperation.

'You are so ugly, no one is going to want you,' he replied.

'Go away,' I said, turning my back and walking away, every muscle in my body readying itself for the strike that was sure to come.

My father was strict, and inflexible, and I was already tired of his antics. He was quick to anger, quick to use his fist, and not only had I started to accept that the consequences were predictable but also that I was prepared to face them. I was an excellent student. I consistently topped my exams and the school year. I played national-level sport. I woke every morning at 6 a.m. to iron all our uniforms and make my parents' morning coffee. I could not understand why my father was so angry.

* * *

In complete contrast to her cantankerous husband, my mother was happy and giving. Laughter was her medicine, and, in the 1980s, so was the music. She sported the perm and shoulder pads that proved her commitment to Whitney, one of the greatest voices of all time.

My mother was 21 years old when she had me. I remember the smell of biscuits when I came home from school, and watching her teach herself to drive from our front window when I was five, maybe six. When she finally mastered it, she would drive me to the corner store a few times a week, and we would eat ice cream together, just the two of us, protected by the bubble that was the inside of the car.

Food was her love language. She gave it to all those around her in a memorable way. One day, we found her over the stove, stirring a large pot. She was seasoning it carefully, tasting it to make sure it was acceptable. She decided it needed a little extra salt. 'Who is this for?' we asked, and she replied, 'It's for the dogs.' We laughed, mistaking her rapid answer for a joke, although such a joke would not have been to her taste. 'Well, dogs enjoy good food too!' she admonished.

Her culinary prowess and love of good food also lent itself to the role of food critic. One day, having painstakingly slaved away in the kitchen for an entire afternoon to prepare dinner for her and the rest of the family, I proudly set the table, dished up her meal and waited for her nod of approval. My mother sniffed it first, as she always did when someone else had cooked, then said, 'Did you put enough pepper and onions in this? Because it smells like underarms.' I was infuriated, and regretted immediately the effort I had made to impress her.

Nonetheless, I loved to be with my mother. If she was leaving in the car, nine times out of ten I was in the passenger seat. If she was cooking in the kitchen, I was there helping her. As I cut onions for her one day, she scolded me for speaking ill of someone I had seen earlier. 'Always be kind to those around you. You never know when you might cross an angel,' she said gently. This culminated in me wondering if every bug I squashed, every mosquito I slapped, might also be an angel.

My capacity to work is undoubtedly a gift from my mother. Her paternal grandfather was Chinese, and settled in Samoa in the 1890s when Chinese labourers were migrating to the Pacific Islands to work on the plantations. I am sure this cultural heritage is very important and was a key reason for my mother's work ethic, and that of all her sisters and brothers. She started her catering business when I was 13 years old, and quite quickly became known on the island for her delicious cooking. I remember waking at two o'clock in the morning to harsh light in my eyes and the horrible sound of the eggbeater. I would lie in bed for as long as I could before ultimately deciding to get up and help her. At that hour, she would be making her custard pies, and my job was to press the bases into the aluminium moulds. I did this until my fingers hurt and I could do no more. My mother would work non-stop until late in the night, and sometimes I would catch her crying with fatigue and exhaustion. Two o'clock in the morning will always be my mother's hour. That is when she would wake and start to work.

As children, we spent a lot of time with my mother's family. My maternal grandmother was devoutly Mormon, and would spend days fasting and praying for each of her children and grandchildren. Every time our exams rolled around, our grandmother would pray and fast for us. Every time a member of the extended family had something important happen, or was unwell, she would pray and fast. Caring for the larger family unit was important, and we spent many evenings, lunches and Sundays sharing meals with one or several or all of my mother's 13 siblings and their mother. While there was a lot of laughter among the aunts, uncles and cousins, everyone also loved sports and competition. Family volleyball often ended up with manhandling and arguments, as an aunt or uncle took it upon themselves to push one or all of the other players aside to return the ball over the net.

My paternal grandfather lived alone, his house atop a mountain, watching over the capital of Samoa. He would walk down the mountain to our house, barefoot on the dirt road, carrying only a rifle, and on arrival would want only a cup of coffee. He would take his coffee to the balcony at the back of the house, light a cigarette and sing 'How Great Thou Art' at the top of his lungs. One day, as I sat next to him, he imparted some grandfatherly wisdom: 'Do not let anyone touch you here.' He pointed to his own groin.

* * *

My first foray in the Samoan public hospital was at the age of 15. Actually, it was six years earlier than that, after I had been bitten by dogs on the side of the road, but back then I had only needed antibiotics injected into my glutes. This time, I had taken my parents' car and somersaulted it into a cemetery.

My parents were in New Zealand, and had been for the couple of months prior, because my mother was pregnant with her sixth child and, if one can afford to scrape the money together to travel to New Zealand or Australia for medical care, this is the ideal. Well-trained doctors and compassionate nurses were a little lacking in Samoa at that moment in time. The nurses were known to scold a woman in labour who might cry or moan through contractions. 'Be quiet!' or 'Did you think it was supposed to be pleasurable?'

were the reprimands whispered between women who had delivered their children at the national hospital.

On the same day my mother gave birth to my youngest sister, I had decided to take the car, some friends, a few surfboards, and head to the beach. I had been driving from the age of about 13, and at the age of 15 got my licence by handing $20 to a police officer and passing a test that required island logic. If you drive through a village and hit a child, do you a) stop to help, or b) keep driving? The correct answer was b). The practical part of the test was not much less of a trap. 'Pull over here! Right now!' the policeman ordered, as I drove at an appropriate speed with my hands at two and ten o'clock. 'Now! Pull over!' he insisted, as I slowed the car and put it into neutral perfectly parallel to the sidewalk. 'Why did you stop here?' he said. 'This is a bus stop! You should not have stopped. You fail this part of the test.' Logic and sensibility were not always evident, but if one was resilient enough the system could be worked around.

However, when I wrote my parents' car off and found myself responsible for broken limbs and cuts and scrapes but no death (as was so common among youth in traffic accidents), I considered myself lucky. I could not ruin my life, or the life of another.

* * *

When my parents returned from New Zealand with their sixth child, their relationship took a turn for the worse. My mother had departed for New Zealand early in her pregnancy, to start timely antenatal care, but my father had only joined her weeks before her due date. In the months that he had been alone, he'd had an affair, and everyone on the small island had come to know of it. On her return, so did my mother.

It was around this time that my relationship with her changed. I started to take a more protective role, and my mother would confide in me the way one might confide in a friend. Our evening rides in the car, which had ten years prior been escapades for ice cream, evolved into evenings where she would express her disappointment and confusion over what had happened. I did not enjoy these discussions. Frankly, it did not please me to hear the details, but I realised my mother was fragile, hurt and alone, and she needed support in a new way.

As I drove along the main road in town, the sea on one side, the restaurants and nightclubs on the other, I would feel a sense of doom. I realised that I could not stay. As beautiful as it was growing up swimming in waterfalls, rivers and the sea, there was no future here that I could see. The monotony of life frightened me. Friends married other friends, and frequented the same bars and nightclubs in their thirties as they had in their teens.

By the time I was 15, there were six children in the family, and it seemed that it was going to be each of us for ourselves. My two best friends had left for boarding school the year prior, and I begged to be sent too, but my parents simply could not afford it. There was no possibility that my parents would be able to afford to send me to university overseas, either. So, I worked. When my friends were out, I studied secretly, happy in the knowledge that I was working while they were not. I knew that this was how I would get ahead. At 17 years old, I won a fully paid scholarship to study medicine in New Zealand.

When people ask why I did medicine, the simple truth is that it was my path to freedom. There were only a few scholarship awards to New Zealand at that time, and unfortunately aviation school was not one of them. They were classic vocations such as medicine, law and accounting. I chose medicine because it gave me a flight and a future beyond the islands. My only regret was that my mother could not leave with me.

* * *

It was a requirement of the university that, as an entrant from the Pacific Islands, I spend the summer attending an English course. Despite the fact I could speak fluent English and had been educated entirely in English, I was forced to pack my bags just after Christmas and spend two months being 'taught' English again. I lived with a homestay family: a middle-aged woman with a well-advanced diabetic foot ulcer, her husband, and her brother, who had schizophrenia. It was a rude awakening, far away from the home that I thought I had been ready to leave behind me. Here is where I learnt that some people eat dinner at 5.30 p.m.

Two months later, I started enrolment. This required that I circulate through all the basic science departments to obtain their approval. Judging from the responses I received – which included 'Where did you learn to speak English so fluently?', 'Do they have electricity in Samoa?' and 'You are going to struggle to make it through these papers' – they did not think very highly at all of high-school graduates from Samoa, even though our curriculum was based on the New Zealand high-school curriculum.

And, once my enrolment in a pre-medicine year was approved, I proceeded to fulfil their expectations. I was homesick and miserable, longing to be close to my mother, and increasingly disappointed that she stayed in a marriage in which she found little joy. I scraped through the first year of medicine, then failed the second, and received a letter telling me I was going to lose my scholarship and must present for an interview. That was my wake-up call. I could not go back. I studied like a demon over Christmas, re-sat the exams in the New Year, nailed them, and promised myself I would never let that happen again.

* * *

Three years later, in my fifth and penultimate year of medical school, I went to Austria and Italy to do an elective in orthopaedic trauma. I'd chosen orthopaedics because, as is often the case, I'd worked with a professor who'd inspired me while I was a student. I travelled nearly 24 hours to arrive in Innsbruck, and when I found myself sleeping up to 14 hours a day, I thought it was jetlag, but then my nipples started hurting. It was the middle of winter, and the temperature during the day was −5°C. I had never been in a place where the temperature dropped below zero. I decided that the breast and nipple pain was due to the cold. For three months, I continued to explain my symptoms away, but once I was back in New Zealand I made an appointment to see my doctor.

'Could you be pregnant?' he said nonchalantly.

'Absolutely not,' I replied. The idea that I could be pregnant had not crossed my mind. I had, however, been eating about ten apples a day and my breasts were fuller. Someone had called out to me on the street about them, which had never happened in my life, and one of the doctors at the hospital had said there were comments about my 'décolletage'. I had never in my life had a problem with décolletage, unfortunately, so I found the remark completely insulting.

'Let's just do a pregnancy test to make sure,' my doctor said.

I knew this game in a tired female of reproductive age, so I conceded. He added beta-HCG to the laboratory form and sent me to have a host of blood tests that would be routine for a young woman complaining of tiredness. I was not prepared for his call later that afternoon.

'You are pregnant,' my doctor said bluntly.

I was shocked. A thousand thoughts flew through my head, but I could not grab any one of them. 'I cannot have a baby,' I said.

'I thought you might say that,' he replied calmly. 'I have booked you an ultrasound scan on Monday to date your pregnancy, and I have spoken to my obstetrician colleague who can tentatively pencil you in for a termination on Thursday.'

It was a Friday. The day that I found out I was pregnant was a Friday.

'Your scan on Monday is at 10 a.m. I suggest that you do not look at the screen,' he continued. 'Let's talk again on Monday afternoon.'

I was surprised that he had organised all this in advance, but he had known me for years, and I was grateful for the immediate path in front of me.

I spent the weekend floating around the house like a ghost, but reassured there was a plan in place. I was no longer with the father, and I had a big year ahead. As well as being in the final year of medicine, I was also part of the Samoan Netball World Cup team, and had been training intensely in preparation for travelling to Jamaica in three months' time.

On Monday morning, I presented to the clinic for my dating ultrasound, and did as my doctor told me, closing my eyes and avoiding the screen altogether. 'Oh, look at those arms and legs,' I heard the radiographer say. 'And that little heart.' I opened my eyes and saw that there was indeed a well-formed little human on the screen, with four limbs and a heart with chambers, just like we had studied in medical school.

'Fuck,' I whispered, my heart racing.

'You are twenty-six weeks pregnant,' the radiographer said matter-of-factly. 'Congratulations.'

I was in a state of shock. I knew what 26 weeks pregnant meant. It meant that I had only 14 weeks of being pregnant left. It meant that I was going to have a baby in my last year of medical school.

'There are places in Sydney where you might be able to have a termination,' my doctor said to me over the phone that afternoon. 'Or we can look at options for adoption.'

'No,' I replied.

I believed that everything happened for a reason, and the late discovery was a gift. I had never wanted to have children. After watching my mother raise six of us, I had long crossed it off my list, and had big plans to move to the other side of the world as soon as I possibly could. But I accepted that, perhaps, this was on my path after all, and I had the malleability to ride it – and I quickly moved on to the next stage of planning.

'Refer me to a good obstetrician?' I asked my doctor.

I was already mentally calculating exact gestational dates, training dates and my departure date for Jamaica. My due date was the end of July, so if I had a caesarean section at 36 weeks, that would be end of June … and maybe I could even push that to 34 weeks, which would give me a few weeks to recover and still play in the world cup. I was determined. I was 22 years old, and I did not see that I would have the opportunity to play again.

'Don't be ridiculous,' the obstetrician said when I explained my plan to him. He was tall, a little overweight, balding and not inspired by my passion. 'There is absolutely no way you can do that,' he said. 'And you have to stop running. You are overheating your baby and, actually, you don't have a lot of amniotic fluid, so we need to keep an eye on you. You might need to be on bedrest.'

A door slammed shut. Jamaica was over. I was going to be a mother in July and, all going according to plan, a qualified doctor in December.

* * *

In a twist of fate, I was attached to obstetrics and gynaecology while all this was happening. I returned to class later that same day and learnt all about the stages of labour. I walked out of that class probably looking a little dazed and confused. I had not told a soul what was happening.

A friend followed me out of class. 'Are you okay?' she asked.

Evidently, I was not doing a great job at pretending that everything was normal.

'I'm twenty-six weeks pregnant,' I told her, surprising myself. Even when I had gone to school with my eyes swollen from crying the morning after a hiding from my father, I would tell people I had slept on my front.

'Have you told your mother?' my friend asked.

'Nope. Not a soul.'

'You should tell your mother,' she said. 'She will be disappointed to miss out on this.'

My friend did not know my mother, but I had not thought of it this way. That night, I called her. She was ecstatic, absolutely thrilled, and immediately made plans to fly over and help with preparation for the last few weeks of pregnancy, and would stay on for a couple of months after the birth.

My father? He stormed out of the house after demanding that I get married, because there was no way that he wanted a bastard grandchild.

* * *

Fourteen weeks of pregnancy rolled by rapidly, and reasonably calmly, as I set about readying myself to be a mother in medical school. I wanted my transition into motherhood to be seamless, and I wanted to graduate from medical school in six months' time.

I was living with two of my sisters and my brother, and they were going to be part of my 'village'. When my mother flew in two weeks prior to my due date, she took pleasure in buying the essentials for a newborn baby. She was with me in the delivery suite, and she stayed by my side for eight weeks after the birth. Then, she had to get back to her own life.

I gave birth on a Monday, and four days later – on Friday – I returned to my paediatrics rotation to sit the exam the department had not allowed me to postpone. I passed with distinction.

Then, the following Monday, I started my rotation in general practice. Armed with a supply of bra inserts to soak up the milk that was leaking from my breasts, I sat in the clinic listening to rattly chests and looking at infected ears. My baby boy stayed at home with my village. And, with their support, I graduated five months later as a doctor.

2.

Do the best you can until you know better

I spent my second year as a junior doctor – also my second year as a single mother – working as an emergency doctor throughout Australia, wondering if I would be happy in such a specialty. It allowed me to travel, and as I moved from one Australian beach town to the next, I thought it had all the makings of a cool lifestyle. However, after a year of seeing young women with urinary tract infections, children with cockroaches in their ears, dental abscesses because of lack of access to good dental care, and a friend destroyed because he misdiagnosed a patient with a near-fatal result, I returned to New Zealand to start specialty training in … something else.

I landed in urology, and developed a passion for foreskins and prostates. I enjoyed both the specialty and the weird personalities that practised it. I particularly adored the head of department at the time. He was a little unconventional, brilliant but strange. We would find him sitting in the tearoom on the ward before seven-thirty in the morning, which was neither usual nor necessary, as the ward rounds were normally run by the senior registrars and did not require the consultant surgeon also.

'What are you doing here so early?' I asked him one day. 'You don't need to be here.'

'The house is too noisy and the kids are all over the place, so I told my wife I had to come to work,' he offered as he flipped through the latest issue of *Cosmopolitan*.

'Shall we go then?' I prompted him to stand and round with us.

We meandered to the first cubicle.

'Oh, fuck,' he muttered, then pulled me out to explain the 'situation' (aka the patient). 'This old guy has balanitis, and he needs a circumcision,' he said. 'It's a shame, because he's got a big dick ... but he's ninety and doesn't use it anymore. Anyway, his carers are upset, so can you just tell them he is booked for theatre? Thanks, buddy.' Then he pushed me back through the curtains, leaving me to deal with the situation while he waited for me at the exit of the ward.

It was funny, but it was also the right thing to do. Not all surgeons are gifted communicators, and this urologist – though brilliant – was not known for his bedside manner. As a surgical registrar, you soon realise that one of your roles is mediating the relationship between patients and your consultant. We would laugh about how this particular supervisor would push us through the curtains and hide behind them, but in fact we communicated better than he could. And, in this instance, he wanted me to explain the problem to the patient and his carers: the man's foreskin was inflamed and, after multiple episodes of inflammation, the foreskin around the tip of the penis was so scarred and tight that it had closed the meatus, barely allowing urine to pass through. Circumcision meant this would never happen again. After reassuring the patient and his carers, I left, closing the curtains behind me.

My supervising urologist had incredible general knowledge of the world — we would find brainteasers that Microsoft and Google used for their technical interviews and do them together, and you could ask him anything — but he would distress patients. 'You need the catheter in for three weeks,' he told one patient, who also happened to be the father of a close friend in medicine, on day two after a major cancer operation. My supervisor was standing at the end of the bed and holding four fingers up. 'Three weeks. Okay, buddy? Three weeks.' Again, with his arm stretched out in front of him, he held four fingers up. Then a thumbs-up. And exit left.

'What on earth?' the patient breathed, looking around in disbelief.

I tried to reassure him. 'Surgery went very well. You look exactly as you should for day two post-op, and you will probably go home tomorrow, okay?'

Not infrequently, I would feel that managing my supervising surgeon was like managing a child.

* * *

My own son was three years old when I started in these surgical specialties, and it was just the two of us. He had spent the previous two years living with my mother in Samoa – an arrangement she had suggested, as he was her first grandchild and she wanted him close to her. But, after two years of living apart, it was too hard. I brought him back to live with me.

My days were long. I had to leave the house at 7 a.m. to get to ward rounds, and had night shifts interspersed with day shifts. But no daycare facility opened early enough or closed late enough to be useful and, more importantly, my heart broke leaving my son there for such long days – I'd have to wake him before sunrise to get ready in a mad rush and be at work on time. I decided it would be kinder for both of us to have someone living at home. So, I sponsored a relative from Samoa to come over, live with me, help with his care and cook for us.

The guilt never stopped. Guilt for choosing a specialty that compromised our time together, guilt for leaving so early in the morning, guilt for coming back so late at night. But I was on the train, and I was addicted to the drama, the work stories and the mess. As long as I could keep all the balls in the air, I would keep going.

That winter, my son was endlessly unwell, as three-year-olds who go to daycare tend to be. One morning, I arrived home after a long night on call as the surgical and urology registrar to find him looking miserable. He had been unwell with a cough and runny nose, but was going to stay home from daycare with the relative, so I curled up under the sheets and fell asleep. When I woke, it was 8.30 p.m., and I had to leave again for the hospital in an hour. I found my son on the couch, breathing rapidly, looking flushed and unhappy. I gave him an 'objective' mother's once-over, meaning I lifted up his shirt to clarify how hard he was working to breathe. He had indrawing: every time he took a breath in, his soft skin and the muscles in between the ribs were pulled inwards. It is a sign of respiratory distress, and my heart stopped to see his little chest working so hard. I quickly changed, wrapped him up in a blanket and took him in the car to the hospital, wondering at the same time if I would be able to leave him in the emergency department overnight while I did my night shift.

I had only dropped two enquiries with the nursing staff when the consultant on duty in the emergency department took me aside. 'You have the right to call in sick to look after your son,' he said. 'Don't leave him in the emergency department alone.'

I called in sick and felt sick doing so.

* * *

It was during my time on urology that I learnt that foreskin education is particularly important for young men. I realised I would have to educate my son about caring for his foreskin – cleaning it, making sure he could roll down the prepuce and be sure that it was not forming a tight band (balanitis). I would also have to make sure that he knew that, when he rolled it down, he should clean it. But most importantly, he must always pull back the foreskin over the head of the penis again ... Okay, fine. I am a little obsessive.

As my son was born during my final year at medical school, we really lived our formative years somewhat in parallel: me, in surgical training; him, in early adolescence. Unfortunately for my son, I think these years were much more traumatic for him than they were for me, especially after intrusive conversations like the one above. But these particularly important life lessons for a young boy were reaffirmed in my work as a junior registrar in urology – and, whenever they were, I patted myself on the back for being a good mother. (It did not happen often.)

One day, I was called to the emergency department to see a patient in his late twenties with what is called a paraphimosis. Let's call him Mr L for Lizard. (You will understand why.) Paraphimosis is considered a urological emergency, and the whole affair can be dramatic. You see, this is a condition that occurs in uncircumcised men and happens when the foreskin is retracted behind the glans penis, also known as the head of the penis. The foreskin becomes swollen and constricted behind the glans penis, such that it can no longer be rolled back over the head of the penis. At its worst, it can be so constricting that it slows or stops blood supply to the tip of the penis. And, while it sounds extremely dramatic, it looks even worse. Think frilled-neck lizard.

Twice in my life I have seen paraphimosis in young men occurring after sexual intercourse – another important life lesson to impart. Always pull the foreskin back over the head of the penis after sexual intercourse. Mr L was one of the two. After having sexual relations with his girlfriend that evening, he'd been alarmed a few hours later to find his penis looked grossly abnormal. He was mortified. So was I. We were around the same age. One could imagine that we might have crossed each other on a night out. What he did not know was that I was about to spend the next 30 minutes with my hand firmly gripped around the head of his penis. Unfortunately, unless he was to have an acute circumcision, the non-operative management is – for want of a better word – awkward. (Circumcision is the last resort if non-operative management fails.) This young man and I were about to become intimate friends.

I set about readying my trolley: lignocaine jelly to numb the foreskin, a needle, gloves, my hand, and lots of small talk. Check, check, check, check and check. Swallowing my rising alarm, I applied the numbing jelly to his foreskin, which was becoming more and more swollen in front of our eyes. Then, I took my needle, apologised profusely, and stabbed his swollen foreskin multiple times around its circumference. This helps to get rid of the excess blood and fluid, and you don't always need to do it, but it makes the next and most awkward step shorter (and, believe me, it still feels as if it is taking a lifetime, even when you use the needle).

Once I was happy with the needling, I apologised again, then wrapped my hand around his penis and squeezed. Really squeezed. There is no other way. 'Mr L, could you shuffle over on your bed so I can sit on the edge?' I asked. 'I'm going to be here for a while.' And so, with my hand wrapped around his penis and his leg against mine, we shared that small hospital bed, and started to chat.

There is a lot you can talk about during this time. The weather, university, family, favourite sports, pets, life plans, religious views, political affiliations ... You get the picture. Finally, his penis co-operated, and we were done before the end of the night. Mr L walked out of the emergency department with a bruised ego, and my fingers imprinted between his legs.

Another cautionary tale, and another note-to-self: tell my son to pull his foreskin back not just after a shower or peeing, but also after sexual intercourse. This would follow rules one and two: don't open the door to anyone when I am not home, and don't call me unless there is an emergency.

* * *

Waking up to pee in the middle of the night becomes increasingly problematic for men of a certain age. They can thank the prostate for this.

The prostate is a small gland the size of a ping-pong ball that sits at the base of the penis and below the bladder. From the age of about 25, the prostate starts to grow slowly and, by virtue of its location, can cause symptoms consistent with obstruction of the bladder. This includes difficulty starting to pee, a poor stream, a frequent need to pee and difficulty emptying a full bladder. Commonly, because of an enlarged prostate, men present in acute urinary retention, meaning that they cannot pass urine despite the desperate urge to do so. If there has been bleeding into the bladder because of the superficial vessels over an enlarged prostate, this can lead to haematuria (bloody urine) and therefore clot retention. This means that blood clots cause obstruction to the outward flow of urine. This is managed with a two-way urinary catheter for irrigation of fluid into the bladder and flow of urine out. The haematuria is described according to how blood-stained it is: rosé haematuria, shiraz or cabernet merlot. The closer to rosé it is, the closer a man is to going home with or without a catheter.

A 68-year-old man presented to the emergency department in acute urinary retention. He was in distress. He had not been able to pass urine for most of the day, and was experiencing both lower abdominal pain and an intense urge to pee. Examination was consistent with a grossly distended bladder, and I told him I would have to insert a tube through his penis into his full bladder to drain it. 'After that, you will feel so much better,' I promised.

I washed my hands, donned a pair of gloves, gave his penis a wash with antiseptic solution, inserted some lubricating jelly with lignocaine into his penis (to both lubricate and anaesthetise), and then inserted a catheter. It sailed smoothly in … until it reached the prostate. Then, it would not budge.

'No problem,' I said, then reached for a wider catheter from the trolley. Sometimes, if the prostate is bulging into the urethra, it requires a wider, more rigid catheter to traverse the base of the bladder. The diameter of a urinary catheter can be small (a size usually reserved for females or children) or large, or even very large. The very large catheters are stiff, and we use them for difficult catheterisations. Unfortunately, this did not work. Next in the line-up was an introducer, which looks as if it is made from a manipulated wire coathanger. But not even loading the catheter onto this contraption could convince the prostate to allow me across. By this point, my patient was thoroughly unimpressed and desperate for relief.

I had one last resort: direct access through the abdominal wall and into the bladder. I took a new instrument trolley, cleaned his lower abdominal wall directly over the top of the bladder, chose a scalpel to incise a two-centimetre window through the skin, then plunged a trocar directly through the muscle and through the bladder wall until I got urine. And I got urine. The bladder, under pressure with 1.8 litres of fluid, exploded through the trocar. I ended up on my back foot trying to grab a catheter bag, as a 2007 shiraz rained down on our heads. It was almost biblical, but I kept my mouth closed.

After letting out a profound sigh of relief, my patient looked around the room and at the floor. 'It looks like a murder scene in here,' he said.

I had to agree.

* * *

It was not for murder but certainly as an instrument of communication that I came to rely on these urinary catheters. As the most junior of the urology team, I was delegated the least enviable task: running the catheter clinic.

This is where men or, on the rare occasion, women who had gone into urinary retention would present with their catheter for what we called a TROC – a trial removal of catheter. It was quite simple. The catheter would be removed, the patient would be asked to drink a couple of litres of water quite quickly, and then, once they had the urge to urinate, they were encouraged to go to the toilet. If they could pass urine, it was a win. If they could not, they required another TROC at a later date, medication or surgery.

Unfortunately, as would be the case, there were two or three 'clients' who enjoyed attending the catheter clinic far too much. They would book themselves in a little too frequently. One day, as I was leaving the ward, my son in tow, one such client was waiting at the exit. I was surprised to find Mr BS there, said hello, then tried to quickly walk past him, but he jumped into the elevator with us and persisted with questions about our lives. Before the elevator stopped on the ground floor, he handed me his business card.

'You are very pretty,' he said. 'You will do well in private urology, and you should call me when you have your practice.'

I hurried out of the elevator, clutching my son's hand, disgusted.

The next day, the same client turned up, insisting on having yet another TROC. Unimpressed, I commenced him on his TROC pathway – catheter removal, and two litres of water to drink – and at the end of the day the nurse called to say he needed another catheter.

'Get the 18Fr and 20Fr ready for me, please,' I asked the nurse. These are the big ones.

Mr BS stiffened as his catheter was replaced, but not in the way that he had hoped. He realised this new catheter was notably different from the last. He did not come back the next day.

* * *

Trauma is the main reason to turn up at the emergency department following a sexual-activity mishap, according to a study conducted by Pfortmueller et al and published in the

Emergency Medicine Journal in 2013. Usually, these patients are young men in their twenties and thirties with a fractured penis, excoriated penis and balls, or foreign bodies inserted in places they shouldn't be.

I have seen a few drive-by drop-offs, where partners have left patients at the front door without so much as a kiss goodbye. Mr BP (for broken penis) got a kiss goodbye, and he got me out of bed. He had been having sex with his girlfriend and decided, in a moment of passion, to pick her up and pin her against the wall. It looks good in the movies, right? Unfortunately, gravity always wins. She fell and crushed his penis at an awkward angle, and the immediate and severe penile pain saw her load him straight into the car. Before she left after dropping him at the front door of the hospital, she meekly told the triage nurse his penis looked like an emoji – the eggplant one.

I was thrilled. I had never seen a penile fracture before. I made sure my son was fast asleep, then asked the neighbour to be 'on call' for him in case he woke, and raced into work. Training in surgery was an exciting journey. A hunger for stimulation was fed by things we might see once in a lifetime, or by the madness of what people might do to themselves. Most of the time, it was rewarding. In the operating theatre that night, I was blissfully rewarded as I watched the urologist skilfully open Mr BP's broken penis, evacuate the haematoma, and suture the broken layers back together again.

Mr BP was discharged the following day with strict instructions to refrain from sexual intercourse for at least six weeks.

* * *

After three months of urology, I had decided well and truly that emergency medicine was not for me, but I took extra duties where I could, and had taken an extra shift as the junior registrar on night duty in the emergency department. In training, you can't always get the good. Sometimes, you head home after a shift feeling demoralised. This was one such time.

There were two other senior registrars on duty, and we were swamped with patients. It was a Friday night, and a fairly typical one at that. All the patient cubicles were full, and patients were being assessed on trollies in the corridor. Chest pain and traumas were rolling in one after the other, and then a sixteen-year-old girl was brought in by her family after an attempted suicide.

I was called over the department intercom to see her in resuscitation bay two. When I arrived, she was lying on her side, and the nurses were trying to get an intravenous line in to take blood samples and give her fluids. She was a robust girl, not at all small, so inserting a needle into one of her veins was difficult even for the experienced nurses. Her mother was there, and her four sisters. I heard them speaking in Samoan as I entered the room.

'Is she the doctor? She looks like she still wets the bed,' one of them said, thinking that I could not understand. Apart from such useless commentary, they did not say much unless I asked questions pointedly.

The girl, meanwhile, was breathing spontaneously, but she would not open her eyes. She had a good, strong pulse and a normal heart rate. Her blood pressure, temperature and blood glucose were also normal. So far, so good. There was nothing leaping out as life-threatening to deal with, so I stepped back and asked the girl what she had ingested. She would not respond so, while I attempted to place a large-bore intravenous line into the crook of her elbow, I turned to her mother. 'What did she take?' I asked.

'Augmentin,' her mother replied.

The nurses and I exchanged glances. One rolled her eyes.

'Augmentin?' I said.

'Yep,' the mum replied. 'She took sixteen capsules about an hour ago.'

Augmentin is an antibiotic. The worst thing that could happen was that the girl would have a terrible bout of diarrhoea or contract vaginal thrush. At that moment, as I was still trying to insert the needle into her arm, the girl opened her eyes and, with her other arm, punched me square in the face.

'Ha!' The mother clapped her hands. 'Did she get you good, doc?'

All five girls were chuckling.

The nurses and I were absolutely dumbfounded, but I was not proud of my reaction. I am not proud still. 'Get the fuck out of this department! Get the fuck out!' I shouted.

With that, the girl jumped off the bed, put on her clothes, and joined her mum and her sisters as they ambled out of the department, still laughing.

Of course, it had been the wrong thing to do. For all I knew, she could have ingested something more dangerous than simple antibiotics. I was ashamed as I headed home, and I fell asleep worried that I might have missed something more lethal in the girl's presentation, then woke embarrassed about how I had handled her. Night shifts are hard, and decisions made in the dead of night become doubtful in the harsh light of day, under the scrutiny of fresh eyes that have had the luxury of a night's slumber.

The next day, the head of department asked me to press assault charges. He had spoken to the police and the patient. At least I knew she was alive and well. But I didn't want to press charges. I just wanted the whole affair behind me. A medical student who was a trained and practising psychologist once told me that people should not be blamed for the way they behave when they come into the hospital. I am not sure I agree, because I know that I should not punch my doctor (or anyone!) if I am sick in hospital, but here I felt that I had been in the wrong. I declined to press charges, and instead waited for the week to pass so that I could feel better again.

That was my last shift in emergency.

3.

It will take more than a plaster

I spent two years of my life trying to get onto the urology specialty training programme. Unfortunately, one does not automatically enter their specialty of choice, but must go through an application process that includes research and conference presentations, a skills assessment and an interview. After my second failed attempt, I decided I needed to expand my horizons.

My good friends were in general surgery at the time, and they were endlessly busy. General surgery always had the most patients on the acute operating board, and the most patients to see in the emergency department. There was drama, agitation, mystery and the ability to save a life. It was a beautiful mélange of people, pathology, humour, madness, recovery and loss. In one morning, I could see people from all walks of life. A multitude of stories that made me laugh, exasperated me or left me crushed – the trans woman with acute alcoholic hepatitis that she blamed on Asian soft drinks, the son accusing us of institutional racism over the treatment of his mother, the woman admitted after a round of golf and diagnosed with stage four cancer who did not make it out of hospital, the convicted murderer who did.

I was a convert. And I thought I could do it all. My son was five years old, and I believed that a woman was capable of anything – even being a full-time surgeon and a five-star mother at the same time. Not surprisingly, the lady who had been living with us moved on within six months. My son started flying back and forth between New Zealand and Samoa, spending months at a time in each place before he started school. I was sad for the long separations, but determined to get through surgical training without anyone seeing how affected I was by being a 'non-present' mother. Even more obscene, I tried to get through surgical training without letting anyone know that I desired to be a 'present' mother. I wanted operative cases and I wanted to be a proficient surgeon, and I believed, rightly or wrongly, that if I demonstrated a 'lack of commitment' by having to leave for normal parenting duties I might lose out to the boys. There were no other female trainees at the time. I recall clearly a heavily pregnant senior colleague requesting time off the call roster and being told by a male colleague, 'You are the one who chose to be pregnant!'

I am not sure if it was passion that drove me – although I was passionate about surgery and operating – or if it was the need to prove that I could indeed do it all. My entry onto the general surgical training programme meant relative stability and security as long as I could make it through.

* * *

My son came back to me permanently when he was five years old, and I was happy to have him with me. With my son, my sister and brother had also come back to live with us, and I was grateful for it. I needed my village once again.

I often could not make his parent–teacher meetings, so they had to be done over the phone. 'You need to teach him how to tie his shoelaces,' his matronly teacher scolded me during one.

'Why?' I replied. 'He has Velcro shoes so that he does not need to tie shoelaces. I just don't have time to teach him how to tie shoelaces right now.'

'Yes, but all the kids in class can tie shoelaces except for him. Also, is something wrong at home because he is incredibly moody. He is like a woman who is about to have her period.'

That night, I asked my sister to teach him how to tie his shoelaces.

The next year, I changed his school. He still slept in bed with me, but I did not want that to stop. He was my comfort and, in among all the madness, he was my reason.

* * *

I was in the skin biopsy clinic when an elderly man in his seventies came in with a large and unsightly ulcerated cancer on his bottom lip. The exuberant mass exploded out of the middle of the lip, some 10 to 12 centimetres wide, and it was clear he had not been able to purse his lips for quite some time. Its surface was rough and jagged and oozed blood constantly.

Why he had allowed it to grow so big was a mystery, but we see that sort of thing all too frequently. A woman can present with a large fungating breast cancer that she has wrapped in nappies to absorb the discharge. A young man in the corporate world might present with extensive cavitating abscesses over his buttocks because of a chronic disease for which he has never sought medical assistance. Even stranger, a person's husband or wife, who they have slept in the same bed with every night for years, may be aware of the issue and never have said a word.

This 72-year-old man needed a blood transfusion, because blood had obviously been oozing from the lip cancer for a long time. In addition to that, he drank too much, smoked, lived alone and had poor nutritional status. He was transfused and biopsied. The latter confirmed it was cancerous, which was evident, but we always need a tissue diagnosis. I explained that he would need surgery.

'There is absolutely no way I am agreeing to surgery,' he said without hesitation.

Unable to understand why this dishevelled man whose face was deformed by a removable cancer would refuse, I asked him for the basis of his objection.

'How can I look normal with a big scar in the middle of my face?' he said in complete bewilderment.

I shrugged in equal and absolute disbelief.

* * *

New Zealand has one of the highest rates of melanoma and non-melanoma skin cancers in the world. Australia is the only other country to have a higher rate.

Melanoma is a malignant skin cancer and can be aggressive. Non-melanoma skin cancers include squamous cell and basal cell carcinomas – cancerous growths that occur in the more superficial squamous (flatter) cell layer, or in the deeper basal (round) cell layer of the superficial layer of the skin. They often grow locally, rather than spread, and therefore the treatment is very much based on surgical excision. New Zealand's high rates are thought to be caused by the thinned ozone layer over the country as well as short and intense periods of sun exposure, as opposed to the Mediterranean, where sun exposure is consistent and year-round. The rates are classically highest in Caucasian people. In our skin clinics, most patients are elderly Caucasian farmers or sailors – people who have spent hours, days, weeks, months and years in the sun. Unfortunately, like melanoma, these non-melanoma skin cancers are predominantly found over sun-exposed areas such as the face and ears, and people need multiple skin excisions to take care of little cancers here and there.

I was rostered to cover a skin clinic in a region where a large proportion of the community was farmers. Often, these patients are different from those with a skin cancer in the most expensive beach communities in New Zealand. An 80-year-old farmer, still active and in great shape, presented with a bleeding, ulcerated cancer mid-earlobe. It was bothering him, it was painful, and it was bleeding. He wanted it gone.

Sometimes, if the skin cancer on the earlobe is small enough, we can cut it out, as you would a slice of cake, and then suture the layers back together – cartilage and skin. My assessment said it was just a little too big to do a simple wedge excision, and I was certain that removing the middle third of the man's earlobe – with the cancer in its entirety – would fold the residual earlobe the way you might fold a pancake or calzone.

'I can refer you to a plastic surgeon who will be able to make it look better than I can in a district hospital with just a local anaesthetic,' I told the man, after informing him of my assessment.

He scoffed. 'I couldn't care less what it looks like,' he said. 'I just want my ear to hear and to hold up my reading glasses. I have already waited nearly six months for this appointment.'

The lesion bothered him and caused him pain, and his ear was not at all an instrument of beauty for him. In fact, he wanted it gone. Today. He had other, more important things to do on his farm.

I conceded, perhaps in stupidity, and asked him to lie down on the procedure table. We chatted pleasantly, as I injected the local anaesthetic around his ear. When it was numb enough, I took a scalpel and excised the lesion in two movements: blade across the top, and blade across the bottom.

'It's gone,' I said matter-of-factly, holding the two edges of the remaining earlobe between my fingers, largely to stop it bleeding. People are always surprised at how quick that part is. You can always feel their relief. It is as if to say, 'That was it? What was I so worried about?' I was fairly proud of myself. The man had come in for a service, and I had provided that service. But, as I pulled the earlobe together systematically, suture by suture, I became alarmed at the way it was looking. It was bad. I had not exaggerated when I'd told him it would fold over like a calzone. This is exactly what it did – it looked like a horrible calzone. I nipped and tucked and nipped and tucked to no avail. I hated it. Perhaps he would have been better with no earlobe at all, I thought.

'I'm not happy with this,' I said honestly, completely miserable. I stood him up slowly and walked him to the mirror over the wash basin.

'It's good as new!' he said happily, before thanking me profusely.

Embarrassed at how he would look walking out of the procedure room with a deformed ear thanks to my handiwork, I bandaged it up to cover the evidence. I did not want the next patient to see it. 'Keep that on for the next few days,' I said. 'Hopefully I won't need to see you again.'

His pathology reported clear margins, and I hoped that I would not cross him, or his ear, on the street. I was absolutely mortified by what he (and his family) might think a few weeks down the line.

General surgery has the ability to keep you humble no matter your training or skill level. Before I started the next case, I called a friend. 'Fuck. This poor guy looks like a shark bit his ear,' I exclaimed dejectedly.

'The guy is happy. Don't worry,' he replied. 'And he will still be able to put his reading glasses on.'

* * *

There is a camaraderie in general surgery that's born purely of self-doubt. Did I do something wrong? Did I hurt someone? We train very hard to ensure that we do not.

One day in a surgical handover, a colleague presented a readmission. My good friend, who was sitting next to me, exclaimed, 'Oh no. That's my patient. What did I do now?' He was not negligent at all – I would have trusted him with my own family, and he was well loved by his patients – but it was a perfect illustration of a surgeon's self-questioning tendency. Many of us look through admission sheets to make sure that patients we reviewed the day or week prior have not returned to the hospital or, worse, died. Early in our surgical training, we are taught audit and transparency: we keep logbooks of every procedure performed, we record every complication (minor or major) and death, and we review this frequently with our colleagues to ensure we are operating within best-practice guidelines. Surgical practice should not deviate from 'normal'. These reviews happen in 'morbidity and mortality' meetings, and this continuous audit is an exercise that goes on throughout our careers. What have we done? How many times did we get it right? How many times did we get it wrong? And how do we make it better? Adverse outcomes must be communicated openly with patients, and shared among colleagues.

I was on night shift when an elderly lady presented with vomiting. The emergency department had referred her because she was not settling, and also because it is cruel to send someone home alone at the age of 80. When I assessed her, all her X-rays and blood tests were normal. I could not find anything objective, but I agreed with the emergency department: she was not quite right. So I admitted her, and in the morning told the incoming team about her, expecting she might need some intravenous fluids and would likely get home later that day. Then I went home to sleep.

When I arrived back at work at 10 p.m., I found that she was booked on the emergency board for surgery. She was about to be wheeled into theatre. My heart was racing. What did I miss? I quickly read the acute theatre booking sheet. *Open repair right femoral hernia*. Shit. What an idiot.

I went straight to theatre to find the consultant. 'I am really sorry I missed the femoral hernia,' I told him.

He was washing his hands at the scrub basin, while a few metres away the patient was being drifted off to sleep by the anaesthetist. He turned away from the basin to face me, then said wisely, 'You will never miss it again.'

I appreciated his response. I had expected him to be angry. And he was right. I never missed it again.

After scrubbing in and helping him with the case, I went to the common room, where I found a colleague who was also on night call, but for another surgical specialty. It was midnight by this time, and it was just us two on the couches, watching something ridiculous on the television, waiting for the phone to ring again.

'I missed a femoral hernia last night,' I told him. Sharing our mistakes was a huge part of learning. It allowed us to debrief, find comfort, learn and get up again.

'This is why I left general surgery,' he said. 'At least in vascular surgery, it's definite: either there is a blood-supply problem, or there is no blood-supply problem. But in general surgery, you are always chasing something. I hated to be the guy in the back of the room who missed it.'

He helped me feel better, and when the phone rang for the next assessment I left the common room with my back a little straighter.

* * *

Budding surgeons often learn their basic surgical skills in lumps-and-bumps biopsy clinics. There, they get to use a surgical blade, suture, excise lumps, and put tissue and skin back together in cases that are generally considered to be low risk – you cut out a skin lump and then you close the hole. However, it can still be challenging because, unfortunately, your patients are awake.

It was another Thursday afternoon in the biopsy clinic when a robust Polynesian man presented with a large lipoma on his upper back. For the amateur, a back lipoma is like a lipoma found on any other part of the body … Actually, no, it is not. This is a rookie assumption. Lipomas are benign collections of fatty tissue contained by a capsule underneath the skin that can be felt as a smooth lump, and will often move under your fingers if you put pressure on one edge. On a person's back, however, a lipoma does not move. Nonetheless, it is an obvious lump, and patients might complain about being able to see it under a T-shirt.

Such was the case for this man. He signed a consent form to say he agreed to having an excision of a back lump under local anaesthetic, and then he was placed into position on his stomach. Unfortunately, unlike the beds at a masseuse or a day spa, there is no hole in a hospital bed for you to rest your face in and breathe easily. Nor is the bed softened by a fluffy towel, and there is certainly no relaxing white-noise machine playing the sounds of waves crashing gently on the shore. What I am trying to say is that it is often not comfortable.

I marked out the lipoma. It was quite big – at least ten centimetres – but lipomas usually pop out as soon as you cut through the skin, so the size did not bother me terribly. I infiltrated the local anaesthetic, then once I was confident the area was sufficiently anaesthetised I made an incision directly over it. I had imagined I would cut down on to the lipoma and pop it out the way I had so many times before. No such luck. I could not find a nice, smooth lipoma as I had over forearms or abdominal walls.

I removed my instruments and felt for the lipoma again. It was palpable as a diffuse swelling, and was a little less distinct because of all the local anaesthetic that had been injected. I knew I was in the right place, so I kept going and finally found the lipoma. It was a little deeper than I had anticipated, but it was a lipoma nonetheless. Using scissors, I started to skirt around it as usual. The man winced. As I was deeper than expected, I needed to inject more local anaesthetic. I did so, and waited until he was comfortable, then started again. But the large lipoma was not moving. It was firmly fixed to his back, and the skin was rigid, not at all supple enough to manipulate around the lipoma. I decided to make the skin incision a little bigger to give me better access.

'Can you feel this?' I asked, as I pushed the sharp end of a needle against the skin at one edge of the incision.

'Yes,' he replied.

I injected more local anaesthetic, lengthened the incision, and the exploration continued. He bled as I scissored through the small blood vessels that traversed his fatty tissue. Nothing catastrophic, but enough to be annoying. I asked the nurse to open another pack of swabs to keep the wound dry. Blood was starting to trickle down his sides. I was sure he could feel that his back was incredibly wet.

'You are doing really well,' I said periodically, in an effort to comfort my patient (and myself).

Time was passing, and he was fidgeting on the uncomfortable table. The lipoma was wide and had attachments extending to the layer of fibrous tissue that overlays the muscle. Nothing was freeing easily. He winced again. We were well on to muscle, which was deep in this large man, and everything was stuck. More local anaesthetic, I decided. The problem with local anaesthetic is that there is a limit to how much you can use, and we were fast reaching that point with no sign of co-operation from the lipoma. Meanwhile, the swabs were moving in and out of the field quickly, as they became soaked with blood. This had turned into an ordeal. I could either just close him up and send him home with his friend the lipoma, or I could get help.

'Go grab the consultant,' I whispered to the nurse.

She was as relieved as I was mortified. She was nice, though, because she did not make me feel like I had just made a mess of a very simple procedure.

'Everything is okay. Just a little more difficult than expected,' I reassured my patient (and myself).

The consultant surgeon entered calmly, put on gloves, deftly scissored around the lipoma and delivered it from the wound like a baby. Then we went about stopping the ooze. Simple as that. This happens for years as a surgical trainee. You start a case and, no matter the complexity, you may progress with either ease or difficulty. If it's the latter, you call your consultant, and they breeze in and make it look so easy – so much so, you almost feel ashamed. When one day they arrive and find it just as hard as you, there is a sense of vindication. This particular day was not one for vindication.

'Never do these big back lipomas on this biopsy clinic,' the consultant whispered as I sutured the wound closed. 'They should be done under a general anaesthetic in theatre.'

An hour later, the man, now without a lipoma, was allowed to stand – but only after I had scrubbed away the crusted-over blood that had poured down both sides of his back, and quickly removed the blood-soaked swabs and sheet so he could not see how dramatic it had been. He no longer had a lump visible under his T-shirt, but if he took it off one might see a dent underneath the scar.

I was absolutely exhausted from the stress of the previous two hours. It is definitely much easier when patients are asleep.

* * *

I would run, especially after days like this. The physical exertion cleared my mind and helped me to destress. I was studying for my part-one surgical exam – a little hurdle for all of us on the training programme – and I needed the fracture in monotony before I could sit at my desk and work some more. One summer evening, when the days were still long, I tried to convince my son to join me.

'It is so wonderful to run by the water, to sweat, and to feel that pain in your muscles when it is done,' I said, as I sat tying my shoelaces on the front porch. 'Why don't you want to come?' I wanted nothing more than to have my son share my love of physical activity and sport, but it was turning out to be more difficult than I had anticipated.

'Why would I do something that causes pain and discomfort?' he asked genuinely. It was a valid question. I did not answer him then, but I knew from that moment that our drivers were clearly different. I had worked hard to ensure he would have everything that I wanted as a child but could not have because my parents could not afford it. I traversed pain and discomfort, and wore this like a badge of honour because doing so got me where I was. My son, meanwhile, was gentle because he was raised that way. He did not see the need for pain. We were each a function of our own upbringing.

* * *

I had been living away from home for more than ten years. In that time, my mother had grown a very successful catering business … and my father, who had also launched his own company, was hugely in debt. He had mortgaged everything, including our family home in Samoa, and owed money to multiple different banks. I knew what had been happening and, much to my exasperation, despite the violence and now the debt, my mother still did not leave him.

One day she called me while I was at work. 'The church is undergoing a major renovation, and families can donate money for the windows,' she started.

I could already feel the tension and rage rising inside me, but I remained silent, not inviting what I knew was to come.

'Your dad wants to know if you can pay for the window for our family,' she said.

'How much is it?'

'$10,000,' she replied. 'But the family name will be written on a plaque underneath it.'

'Hell no,' I told her, and hung up the phone.

* * *

Not long after this, I was rostered on call for vascular surgery over the weekend. I was, in fact, the general surgery registrar on call, but at that moment we had to cover vascular surgery and urology also. It can be incredibly stressful to cover other specialties that you are not familiar with, and you spend a lot of time hoping that it will be quiet.

This Saturday did not begin well. If you have to start operating before you finish the ward round, you spend the rest of the day on the run. After a busy morning racing between theatre and the ward, I got a call in the afternoon from a hospital 20 minutes away to inform me a gunshot wound was en route. I was petrified. I was a junior registrar, and dealing with gunshot wounds was not standard fare in our part of the world.

The patient was a convicted murderer who, while out on parole, had taken a gun and gone on a shooting rampage just outside the city. He fatally injured one person and harmed others, before the police shot him through a major blood vessel in his leg. He was being transferred to us because his leg was pulseless, pale and cool, meaning that he would lose it unless it could be fixed. He needed the vascular surgeons to try to reconstitute the blood supply.

At two metres tall and 120 kilograms, he was a formidable man for his size and frightened me even as he lay handcuffed to the hospital bed with a heavy police escort, while I explained the surgery was to try to save his leg. The consultant was going to reroute blood supply from above the injury to a patent section of the vessel below the injury, but restoring this blood supply was not a certainty given the extent of damage. He did not look scared. He was almost leering, and it unsettled me.

The hospital and the ward where he would recover were under heavy police guard, and he was unshaken when he woke up from the first operation, still chained to the bed in ICU. He was equally unshaken when I told him 24 hours later that the salvage had not been successful, and that his leg was dead and needed to be amputated above the knee.

I took him to theatre and fought against his thick, muscly dead leg. It was my first-ever amputation. The consultant had explained over the phone how I should do it, but he did not bother to come in himself. As I sweated and stressed over controlling blood loss and sawing through the bone of the upper thigh, I wondered whether perhaps the consultant might have tried harder to save the leg if our patient had been someone else. We are only human after all. We can't help but feel that some members of society deserve our efforts more than others.

In truth, though, these thoughts were only fleeting, as I paddled upstream, attempting to detach his lower limb. It is usually 'see one, do one, teach one'. Hopefully I would see one soon.

* * *

It was a Wednesday, and what should one do on Wednesday but attempt to be admitted to hospital? At least, that's what this man thought. He was in his thirties and walked through the emergency department doors, unshaven and dishevelled, claiming he had swallowed fish hooks.

Fish hooks? Interesting. Did he have pain? No. Did he have bleeding? No. Did he feel like there was anything stuck in his throat or the rest of his oesophagus? No. How many fish hooks did he swallow? He didn't know. Maybe 20? What made him come to the hospital? He was worried the hooks might cut his insides.

Yes. He swallowed 20 fish hooks before he started to worry. Some people defy logic.

An abdominal X-ray confirmed that he had an abdomen full of fish hooks. We counted 35 around his abdominal cavity, in his stomach, in his small bowel, even in his colon. We admitted him for observation. If the hooks had already reached his stomach, they would probably pass uneventfully. This period of observation entailed daily abdominal X-rays, and daily abdominal examinations in order to detect an intra-abdominal catastrophe early, such as perforation, which he gravely feared. We closely watched those abdominal X-rays and diligently counted every fish hook we could see. Day two: 27 fish hooks. Day three: 22 fish hooks. Day four: 29 fish hooks. (Perhaps the days before they had been lying on top of one another?) Day five: 15 fish hooks. Day six: no fish hooks. They were all gone. Magic.

During his admission we noticed that, when we did the rounds during the afternoon, he was always out. Maybe he was having a smoke. Maybe having a coffee. Maybe drugs. Who knew? But on day six, it was time for him to go home. The fish hooks were out. He was no longer in need of our services.

Imagine our surprise when we arrived on the ward the next morning to find him back in his bed. The exact bed he had just left. The overnight admitting doctor reported that he had come in again claiming once more to have ingested his bag of fish hooks. Sure enough, the abdominal X-ray showed 21 fish hooks, all around his gut and this time including his rectum. A little bizarre that they had moved from his mouth to his rectum within the space of a few hours, but this job teaches you that nothing is impossible.

Not long after our morning handover meeting, a radiographer called us from X-ray to report a wayward fish hook on the trolley. The pieces started to fall into place. Shortly afterwards, an examination confirmed our suspicions. He had been securing fish hooks to his skin so that it appeared on a plain X-ray as if he had ingested them. He had not been swallowing them at all, but rather very carefully attaching them so as to fool us and the simple two-dimensional imaging technology.

It was hard not to admire his ingenuity and dedication to the cause. Moreover, it made me sad to think that he was so lonely he would prefer to be in hospital than at home. He was jovial and in good health, but we often see people coming into hospital because they cannot cope with daily life. There is a special word for this: acopia. Lack of cope. It is known that the elderly Japanese population commit crimes to land themselves in prison for fear of loneliness. This man was not Japanese, but he sure as hell loved his single room on the surgical ward and, apparently, our company. We ordered a psychiatric review for good measure.

One learns over the course of surgical training that there are some problems that cannot be fixed with a surgical blade.

4.

Don't be a
shrinking violet

I had flown to Australia for a meeting when my mother called me in a panic. My father had been complaining of headaches, and that morning had collapsed in church (funny that). Now, he was vomiting. It was not a good collection of symptoms. Even worse, it was not a good collection of symptoms to have where nothing could be done about it.

'Get him on the next plane out,' I told her. He needed a scan of his head without delay.

I organised to fly back from Australia to meet him. I was three years into five years of general surgery training by then, but we had very strict regulations around time off. I found myself picturing the worst-case scenario and how I would manage it. As I landed back in New Zealand, I wondered if I would ever get away from my familial drama. And, when I saw my father, I realised that the answer was probably not. He had a depressed level of consciousness and would stay awake with stimulation only. I waited for the admitting consultant. He walked in with his team, and I sat in the corner, taking up very little space and giving them the opportunity to do their job, which I knew well.

'What made you come to hospital?' the physician asked, and my father's vacant smile demonstrated his inability to reply.

'He complained of a severe headache,' I replied. 'Then he collapsed in church 72 hours ago, and he has been vomiting since.' I worked hard to be pleasantly engaging without demonstrating my distress too much. I wanted to be co-operative, and didn't want to give away that I was medical, as I was aware that it can be difficult to manage patients with family members in medicine. I especially did not want to give away that I could be pushy. I fully recognised that, sometimes, being pushy does not lead to the best medical care.

'When did the headaches start?'

'Several weeks ago.'

'When did the vomiting start?'

'Several days ago.'

'Has he been low in mood lately?' The question surprised me, and I asked the physician to repeat it. 'Is there a history of depression, or has your father exhibited any change of mood in the last months?' he said slowly.

I could feel myself bristling and I tried hard to moderate my response. 'No. Indeed there is not,' I started, but I could not stop. 'However, it seems that he just needs a CT scan of his head. Right?' There, I had said the obvious.

It was the physician's turn to be taken aback. 'We will do a CT scan of the head if it is clinically indicated,' he replied sharply. I would never forget this statement.

I was shocked. 'Well, it seems to me that headaches, vomiting, a collapse and a decreased level of consciousness all indicate an increase in intracranial pressure and a scan of his head is absolutely indicated here,' I said.

Silence.

'Are you medical?' he finally asked.

'Yes, I am a surgical registrar.'

'Well, I think your dad needs a psychiatric assessment. I am worried he could be depressed,' he explained.

'Let me tell you, a Samoan man with a severe headache, vomiting and a decreased level of consciousness does not come to wait in a public hospital with depression,' I said. 'And, the last time I studied depression, I do not think that a severe headache and vomiting was high up on the list of symptoms.'

'You need to let the medical team do what we need to do. We will organise for a psychiatric assessment first.'

I was enraged. I walked out of the cubicle to demand a second opinion, but after a couple of calls to friends who worked in the hospital I decided I would organise for my father to be scanned in a private radiology facility. I knew the public hospital, and I knew it would take several hours before another review because the physicians always have multitudes of patients. Plus, the scan would take hours to organise, and I was adamant this was my father's immediate requirement. Not more reviews. I organised a time for the scan in private care, then went and found the charge nurse for the public ward.

'I have organised a CT scan for my father this afternoon at five o'clock,' I informed her. 'Please can you organise an ambulance transfer to the private hospital?'

'But the psychiatric team are just seeing your father now,' she said.

'I don't care for the psychiatric team to see my father. Please can you ask one of the doctors of the team that saw my father this morning to come and speak with me?'

A couple of hours passed, and a junior member of the medical team popped his head into my father's single room.

'We have requested a CT scan of your father's head. He will be going down shortly,' the young doctor told me.

My father was still incredibly sleepy, waking to pain only, meaning that he would not wake if you shook him gently but he would have if you'd punched him in the guts. The orderly came to collect him, and I accompanied him to radiology. I never knew what the psychiatric assessment found earlier that day, but even with my limited knowledge of neurosurgery I could see that my father had a large haematoma over the left side of his brain – part of it acute and part chronic – and it was sufficiently large that it was pushing his brain against the other part of his skull. He had significant midline shift, indicating that the pressure from the haematoma was important and this haematoma required surgical evacuation. This was the cause of all of his symptoms. He had probably sustained a knock to the head in the recent past, but he now needed emergency surgery.

The junior doctor returned to my father's cubicle an hour later. 'The scan showed a subdural haematoma with midline shift,' he said. 'We have spoken to the neurosurgeons and they are expecting him tonight.'

My father was transferred to the neurosurgical unit, under the neurosurgeon who once looked after Keith Richards (yes, of The Rolling Stones), but I think Keith Richards had a better outcome.

Early the next morning, my father was taken to theatre for a burr-hole (a small hole made in the skull over the fluid) evacuation of the haematoma, and discharged routinely a few days later. After all the drama around getting him to hospital, and getting him to the neurosurgeons, he was in great shape. We were all relieved at the outcome. He would spend a couple of weeks with his sister, before going home to Samoa.

I flew to Wellington to return to work, happy to get back to normal. But a week later, while I was at work, I received a call from a private number. It was the duty consultant in the emergency department. 'Your dad is here. The ambulance brought him in because he collapsed and had a seizure at your aunt's place. We are just working him up, but the neurosurgeons are on their way down. I am just letting you know he doesn't look good.'

My father had a subdural empyema, a major complication after his surgery. The pocket overlying his brain, which had previously been full of a mix of old and new blood, was now full of pus. He was critically unwell and required another emergency trip to theatre. The months that followed are a blur, but he spent weeks in the neurosurgical ICU, with multiple returns to theatre.

Life changed for everyone after this. As for most families when illness (I want to say 'disaster') strikes, everything was turned upside down. Often, as medical professionals, we can forget about the collateral damage to the family in catastrophic illness. Back in Samoa, my mother and sister were trying to take stock of everything my father owed to creditors and the bank, and trying to ensure that the house would not be seized. I called my mother one morning, before his third return to the operating room. 'I am not sure there is any value in you being here,' I told her frankly. 'I think you should just focus on keeping things as stable as possible there.'

She agreed tearily. 'But will you stay close to him?' she asked.

* * *

In between trying to be with my father as much as possible, I'd need to get back down to work, an hour's flight away, so that I could progress through training without delay, but the time spent travelling and waiting by my father's bedside was going to affect my time learning on the operating floor. 'Make me work evenings, nights and weekends,' I told my supervisor. 'I will make up for the time any way possible. I will do extra.'

I was determined to make it through. Getting to the end of training would be freedom for me, and for my son. I had a target date for the end, and I did not want to have to add six months to it. I was also afraid to de-skill in any time that I took off.

Probably because most surgeons have the same bull-headed determination, my supervisor agreed. 'But are you sure?' he asked, after I had spent half an hour convincing him that I was well and the extra work would not be too much at such a stressful moment.

'One hundred per cent,' I confirmed, then supplied all the extra weekend and evening dates I could do.

Thus, I travelled up and down the country with my son in tow. It was a tough time. We spent long hours in the waiting area as my father was put to sleep over and over again. He required multiple returns to theatre for removal of part of his skull and debridement, and then re-debridement. He spent this entire time in the neurosurgical ICU, and we all wondered how this would finally end.

* * *

My mother, not able to stand being away, finally flew over to be by her husband's side. He was not conscious and still febrile, demonstrating that the infection was not yet under control. Furthermore, he had grown multiple hospital bacteria in the microbial culture of his pus, which suggested that he'd acquired the infection in hospital after his first operation. Neither the antibiotics nor his multiple surgeries had been effective thus far in treating him.

One evening, as we sat around his hospital bed – my father was surrounded by his wife and three of his six children – the neurosurgeon came in and informed us they would be taking him back to theatre again the next morning for yet another debridement. He still had a depressed level of consciousness and the infection was not yet under control. 'He likely will not make it,' the neurosurgeon told us. 'He has a high chance of dying from this. You should be prepared.'

We all nodded solemnly, and the neurosurgeon left us to our thoughts. I had not, until that moment, thought of my own parents dying. They were both young, but I already knew that, in the world of medicine, age does not matter. A person can be completely healthy and well one day and gone the next. Medicine teaches you that life is short, and that we should all be grateful for each moment. Nonetheless, it felt surreal that my father could succumb to something 'benign'. I could not accept it. I knew death in cancer and trauma well, but I could not accept that my father would die from this.

My mother cried by his bedside. 'If you make it through this, then we will travel and enjoy life,' I heard her whisper as she took a cold sponge and wiped his feverish forehead.

I was surprised. I had not really considered what losing him might mean for her. Their relationship had been so difficult, but he was her husband and she hoped that their best days were still ahead.

The next morning was my father's last visit to theatre. After that, his temperature started to settle, and just over a week later he started to become more alert. We celebrated. We smuggled champagne and paper cups into the neurosurgical ICU and toasted with him. The acute illness was over, but his life and our lives were different.

At not even 55 years old, my father was finally discharged after several months of brain rehabilitation with headgear that he was to wear permanently. He was epileptic and had lost the ability to speak (dysphasia). You see, the left part of the brain is responsible for speech, and this had been severely impacted by the bleed, infection and surgery. He had lost his independence, his social life, his reason to be.

Nearly a year later, I was in Samoa, rifling through books on our dining table when I came across bits of paper that he had used for his speech and language therapy. The writing was shaky and undoubtedly his: *I should have died.* I was shocked to read this, but I could understand why he had written it. He was in his mid-fifties, fit and well, but he had been handicapped by his dysphasia and epilepsy. He did not have a life.

My mother, meanwhile, had gone back to working double time to pay off the multitude of debts. Those travel dreams she had whispered in his ear when he was unconscious? They were out of the question.

Yes, Keith Richards had a better outcome.

* * *

Teaching in general surgery is a skill. I learnt early that the best surgeons are not only technically skilled but confident enough to let their trainees operate. I was fortunate enough to work with and learn from the best of them.

During a review with my supervising consultants, I asked the lead supervisor not to give me any positive feedback. 'Just tell me what I am doing wrong. I want to be better,' I said, and he laughed.

'I think it's because your father beat you,' a friend said to me jokingly, perhaps not realising the depth of her words.

The next day, I was in theatre, assisting in a very complex surgical case. I was working for an experienced general and vascular surgeon at the time, and he gave me a part of the operation, in the neck, that I had longed to do: I was allowed to suture the carotid artery. He gave me the revered instrument, told me what to do, then scrubbed out. He needed to grab a drink of water, so left theatre momentarily as I started to dissect and suture.

'Why the FUCK are you doing it like that?' he bellowed as he walked back in. Evidently, he had finished his drink of water, and apparently I was working backwards with the sutures more than one and a half millimetres apart. 'Why the FUCK would you make it so difficult for yourself?' he said.

The theatre was quiet, and the nurse across from me muttered under her breath. His theatres were always stressful, and he was known to throw an instrument or two, but we are dealing with people's lives and the stress is maximal for the surgeon whose name is on the bed card. The nurses in theatre with me that day thought he was being a bully, but I felt that I was being taught. I knew I was better for having him as a teacher. Despite his bark, he would scrub in and demonstrate a more efficient or safer way of doing things, and then give back the blade. If you were in trouble and needed help in theatre or out, he had your back.

In training, some of us learnt to deal with situations like that while others did not. I am not sure why. A friend, gifted in surgery, left after an anaesthetist screamed at her and reduced her to tears at the scrub bay before she had even started the operation. She called me in distress, and I found her crying uncontrollably with him yelling at her in front of the entire theatre. We were both young registrars at the time. I asked him to stop, and I told her to leave and compose herself. 'Never let anyone see you crying like that,' I counselled her. I'd had years of training with my father.

Back when I had still been at high school in Samoa, our close-knit group of seven friends had gone out to the local nightclub to celebrate the end of another year. I had finally managed to convince my latest crush to accompany me to the dance floor when I felt a heavy hand grab my hair. Lo and behold, it was my father, and to my utter shame he did not let go. He dragged me out of the nightclub with my head in his big right hand. I was mortified (but my night out had been worth it, as my crush was reciprocated). Now, years later, whenever a consultant would scream at or insult me, or whenever I was shamed in a group discussion for not knowing an answer, I would think that nothing could be worse than my father pulling me out of a nightclub by my hair or striking me down in front of my friends with his right fist. There was no way that I could ever be more humiliated than I had been in those moments. Somehow, it had all ended up being character-building. I certainly did not thank my father for it, but I pitied his inability to be better.

In contrast, I believe in kindness. Specifically when it comes to our jobs and the workplace, if someone is in tears, they are not at their best. We should lift them up. It is our job to empower those around us, no matter our level in training or society. I was bitterly disappointed that my father had never seen his role as that of empowering his wife and his children. The best he could muster was telling me that

I would make a good wife, after I had served dinner one evening.

Outside of work, I would cry at the drop of a hat. To a song (Olivia Newton-John's 'Hopelessly Devoted to You'). To a poem. To a love story. Reading the news. Because someone's dog died. The list is endless. When I watched basketball coach Jim Valvano's speech two months before he died, I adored it. He wisely said that there are three things that we should do every day: 1) laugh, 2) think, and 3) have our emotions moved to tears. I can honestly say that most days I could do all three.

However, if someone was standing over me screaming, berating or bullying, I had been wired not to show emotion. For me, it was important not to demonstrate to anyone that they had broken me. What does not kill you makes you stronger.

* * *

By this stage, I was well advanced on the training programme for general surgery, and I was having a blast. I was surrounded by a good cohort of training registrars and friends, albeit largely male. On the ward, we shared a tiny office that had a single bed I was hesitant to lie on for fear of what happened there. The office was an absolute mess, and probably had been for many years.

'Whatever you do, do NOT clean that office,' my surgeon mentor, who was also a woman, said to me. 'Do not fill that role.'

I was terribly afraid of her. She was strong and said exactly what was on her mind, but later I would learn that she was also sensitive, and loved make-up and clothes. She emailed me when I started surgery with the subject line *Do not be a shrinking violet.* I certainly was not.

When I was in training, I found that there were two types of women to look up to in surgery: those who were supportive, and those who were not. We often said things like 'she is so tough, but she is a product of the old system' to describe a woman who had fought her way through an incredibly male-dominated system and therefore did not have much sympathy for other women who might not have faced the same challenges. On the other hand, there were the women who fought injustice no matter what it was and no matter what they had gone through – in fact, they fought it even harder *because* of what they had gone through. My mentor was the latter. And, once I got over my anxiety that she might think I was a shrinking violet, we became great friends.

* * *

Sometimes, the nights were quiet, and we could sleep in the on-call rooms. Other nights, we did not stop moving. This night was one of the latter. Handover to me was at 10.30 p.m., and already there was at least a page of patients waiting to be seen throughout the wards and in the emergency department.

I settled down with a coffee next to the tray of biscuits, chips and dips that the night staff need to keep quenched and awake. As I ticked off patients who were waiting to be seen, admitting them or discharging them, I received a call from the emergency department staff in a neighbouring hospital 20 kilometres away to say they had an 80-year-old man with a ruptured abdominal aortic aneurysm (AAA). This is a true emergency.

The abdominal aorta is the largest blood vessel in the human body. It carries blood from the heart to the abdominal organs, the pelvis and the lower limbs. When someone has an AAA, which we call a triple-A, it means that the walls of the abdominal aorta have weakened so the aorta bulges like a balloon. This places the individual at risk of the vessel rupturing. The bigger the balloon, the higher the risk of rupture. When it is discovered incidentally – say, because the person has a scan for another reason, or because they have developed abdominal pain – they can either be placed on a surveillance programme, or waitlisted for surgical repair if the risk is deemed sufficiently high. This is based on the size of the aneurysm, and the patient will only be placed on a waitlist for repair if the risk of doing nothing outweighs the risk of doing something.

Nowadays we have options for doing this operation in a minimally invasive fashion, but repair used to be routinely 'maximally invasive', and conducted through a large abdominal incision with all the attendant risks and possible complications. Repair is offered when the triple-A reaches a critical size, and we repair it because, if the vessel ruptures while a person is at home, the chances are it will be a fatal event. Sometimes, a person doesn't know they have a triple-A, and it is only diagnosed when it ruptures.

This particular man did not know he had a triple-A, but he knew he was in trouble. The fact that he had made it to hospital and was still alive was in his favour. However, he was unstable. His blood pressure was low, his heart rate was rapid, and he was sweaty and pale – all symptoms that told us he did not have enough circulating volume. His abdominal girth was growing as blood left the major vessel to accumulate within the abdominal cavity.

The hospital blood bank, which cross-matches a patient's blood type and dispenses blood products, was mobilised for a massive transfusion procedure, and our emergency retrieval team was dispatched to escort him from the neighbouring hospital back to ours. We send a retrieval team if a patient is unstable or risks being unstable during transfer. Massive transfusion protocols are activated whenever massive blood loss is expected and replacing it will be lifesaving, such as in a trauma or a triple-A. One calls the blood bank to inform them, and this starts a regimented protocol for the preparation of red blood cells and other blood products. The man's family – his wife and two sons – arrived before him and were taken straight to theatre, where an anaesthetist was already drawing up drugs and nurses were counting their instruments.

'Let's get the cell saver, lots of packs, and two suctions also,' I whispered to the charge nurse. She already knew we were expecting significant blood loss, and these were standard requirements for such a case. In simple terms, we wanted to reuse the man's own blood if we could with the cell-saver device, which suctions blood from the surgical field, washes the red blood cells, then reconcentrates them for auto-transfusion. We would also have to be able to see what we were doing, so we needed big suckers and lots of packs, because the bleeding can be rapid. The assistant holding the sucker is often the target of fury in these operations. 'SUCK!' the surgeon will say. 'I can't see a fucking thing. SUCK!' (Often followed by, 'I can't see through the sucker. Get your sucker out of the way.')

I explained the gravity of the situation to the family. With a triple-A, every minute of delay matters, and time was passing. Even if the man arrived in the theatre alive, there was a significant risk he could die during surgery, and after that there was at least a 50 per cent risk of death in the 30 days following surgery. The family understood. As he was rolled into the theatre attached to various monitoring machines, blood products and his escort team, his family grabbed him tightly to say their goodbyes – possibly their final goodbyes. They put their heads against his, and told him how much they loved him. Then nothing else was said as they cried over what might lie ahead, or what might not.

Sometimes, in the heat of the moment, these stories pass us as medical staff by, but on this particular night I was hit by the poignancy. While we were moving in the familiar circles of a theatre emergency, this family was holding on to a moment that might never be again.

The man survived his operation that night, and three months later when he came back for a routine post-operative review he thanked us for saving his life.

5.

First, do no harm

Primum non nocere

I completed my general surgical training on a Friday. The weekend passed, and on Monday I walked through the hospital doors as a surgical consultant. It was not quite the caterpillar-to-butterfly transition. I looked exactly as I did the week prior.

Since I was still undecided on my subspecialty of choice, I took a 12-month post as a general surgeon in the hospital where I had just completed my training. There were advantages and disadvantages to this. Advantage: you have established collegial relationships and important supports; they know you and what you are capable of. Disadvantage: they know you and what you are capable of, meaning they know that only last week you were a trainee. I decided the advantages outweighed the disadvantages, and took the post. In my view, I would be able to take on riskier cases knowing I would have ample support.

In a public hospital, there is never a deficit of work, and I was immediately thrown in to seeing patients who had been on waiting lists for months. These were often either patients who had been waitlisted for surgery but their surgeon was unavailable and struggling to keep up with their own urgent cases, or patients who had been waiting just to be seen for a first specialist assessment. It was in this second group of patients that my first challenging operative case as a consultant surgeon materialised.

He was in his late seventies and had been in and out of hospital for months after presenting emergently with a triple-A. This man had survived not only the rupture and the emergency operation to repair the aorta, but also a return to theatre for a relook operation. However, a few months later he was still struggling. Like all presenting complaints, his story was very important. His return to theatre after the first operation had been 24 hours after his emergency aortic repair, because he had been passing blood from his rectum in the ICU and showed all the signs of a colon lacking blood supply – increasing haemodynamic instability necessitating more vigorous blood-pressure support, blood tests demonstrating a lack of oxygenated blood to the gut, and increasing pain-relief requirements.

In a small percentage of patients undergoing elective triple-A repair, there is a disruption of blood supply to the colon. This percentage increases markedly with emergency repair. The corollary of this is that, if the patient survives, the part of the colon that loses its blood supply can die. At the time of this man's return to theatre, it had been felt that his colon was, in fact, viable. So, an attempt was made to restore blood flow by re-joining blood vessels to the affected colon.

Although he had survived these operations, his colon had evidently taken a big hit and the reduction in blood supply had led to severe scarring of the affected gut. He had been suffering because of a severely narrowed left side of his colon, and could only pass small liquid motions and pellets at best. He was near-obstructing and miserable with it, as faecal material accumulated upstream of the narrowing, resulting in bloating, distension and abdominal pain. His quality of life was deteriorating steadily, and he was desperate for someone to help him.

He required surgery to remove the narrowed part of his colon, but elective operating lists for all surgeons in the department were fully subscribed for eight weeks. His last admission with abdominal pain had been two weeks earlier, and the on-call surgeon then had asked if I could assist. Flattered and eager to get my hands on some good operating (in addition to being recognised as an adult surgeon), I said yes. However, he already had two high-risk emergency operations in less than three months under his belt. This was not going to be easy.

Abdominal surgery – or any surgery, for that matter – causes scarring, and I was concerned about how his recent surgeries might add to the complexity of further surgery. If loops of bowel were adherent to each other, or if there was extensive fibrosis and scarring where he had previously had surgery, we risked inadvertently damaging other parts of the bowel, blood vessels or the area specifically related to where we had to re-operate: his left ureter. This is the tube that transports urine from the kidney to the bladder. These were the considerations for entry into the abdominal cavity and resection (or removal) of the narrowed segment of bowel.

The next considerations were related to re-joining the bowel once the resection was complete. Whenever we resect bowel, we aim to re-join it, but we must also consider the safety of doing so. This man was a smoker with diseased blood vessels, which meant that re-joining the bowel ends posed a significant risk of non-healing and a bowel leak. Of course, he did not want to end up with a stoma – when the bowel end is brought to the abdominal wall so that faecal material empties into a bag – but we always keep this as a possibility whenever doing surgery such as this. We held several clinic consultations to talk about the surgery, the possibilities and the man's expectation for recovery. Meanwhile, he was at his wit's end and presenting almost weekly with the unrelenting abdominal pain of the near-obstruction.

With the day of his surgery close, I sought out a colleague to ask if he thought I was stupid for taking on such a case at this infantile moment of my consultancy. I was nervous. I wanted to be brave, but I did not want to be stupidly brave. My colleague's reply was matter of fact: 'If you start in fear, you will always be dictated by it. Have confidence in yourself, and I'll be there if you need me.'

I always had a degree of anxiety on the day of surgery. Perhaps for the small cases, it becomes less stressful, but there are many elements that also make a small case difficult, and it is not uncommon to encounter these same difficulties at every operating list: no assistant, different nursing staff, having to incorporate teaching, the wrong instruments, broken instruments, your list running slow for whatever reason when you are trying to complete a full list. For the larger cases, I would find myself turning scenarios over in my head, planning the roadmap for the approach, making sure I knew what my Plan B was in case Plan A didn't work. This never changes, even after years of being a consultant surgeon. On this particular day in my second week of being a consultant general surgeon, I had considered all possible scenarios, and as the anaesthetist tied up the back of my gown he whispered in my ear, 'You got this.' Having a supportive anaesthetist in a difficult case can change everything. (Sometimes they are not, and this can be horrible.)

As expected, the case was tough. The man was very scarred and the segment of strictured bowel was long. After freeing his adhesions and assessing anatomy, I decided a re-join could not be done safely, and made the decision to bring out a stoma. My colleague from whom I had sought advice came in to give a second opinion, and agreed the stoma was the safest option. The stoma was brought out, I closed the man up, and waited to tell him in recovery. I was surprised by his lack of disappointment. Instead, he was tearful with gratitude that pain might no longer rule his life.

Three months later, after an uneventful recovery, he arrived at the clinic with fuller cheeks. He had finally been able to put on weight, sleep through the night, eat comfortably … and smile. His life had changed.

It goes without saying that the opportunity for this man to be alive, sitting in the clinic with a smile on his face, was owing to at least six months of intensive hospital resource, time, expertise and care from all those involved from the moment the ambulance arrived at his house on day one. His mental fortitude and his trust in us were major factors in his recovery. As for me and my small role in all of it, my surgical colleague and the anaesthetist had given me confidence and allowed me to swim.

* * *

There is often an assumption that surgeons are arrogant, don't really care about their patients as a whole, and operate with disregard for consequences. In fact, surgeons themselves may be responsible for this misconception. In the seventeenth century, Ambroise Paré, a French physician regarded by some as the father of modern surgery, maintained that in addition to 'a strong, stable and intrepid hand', the surgeon must possess 'a mind resolute and merciless'.

Perhaps it is this mercilessness and apparent indifference to making life-or-death decisions under pressure that has since tarnished surgeons with the same qualities as a psychopath. In order to investigate whether psychopaths were indeed over-represented among medical professionals, researchers sent 420 consultants across six hospitals in the United Kingdom a short online questionnaire about the Psychopathic Personality Inventory (PPI), which is employed regularly in the assessment of mental health (Pegrum and Pearce 2015). This assessment tool explores eight subdivisions of the psychopathic personality type, namely: Machiavellian egocentricity, social potency, fearlessness, impulse non-conformity, carefree non-planfulness, blame externalisation and stress immunity. The higher the score on the PPI, the stronger the suggestion of psychopathy. The researchers found that surgeons and paediatricians had the highest scores, and the leading personality traits the surgeons in particular shared with psychopaths were stress immunity and fearlessness. Of course, the diagnosis of psychopathy is only conferred when a candidate scores highly across all *eight* properties of the PPI. Great news.

There are very few publications that investigate the psychological and emotional impact of death on surgeons, but it is without doubt underappreciated (Arnold-Foster 2020; Joliat et al 2019). What we do know is that post-traumatic stress disorder is not uncommon among surgical trainees after a stressful situation. We also know that death places both young and experienced surgeons alike under psychological stress, and puts them at risk of exhaustion and burnout. This is why it is interesting to try to understand where that fictional impression of the detached surgeon arose. Perhaps it was indeed during the era of Ambroise Paré and the barber surgeon when, in addition to providing grooming services for their clients, barbers also conducted minor surgeries and amputations on non-anaesthetised patients.

However, whatever its origins, the detached stereotype today has only negative consequences for both surgeon well-being and patient care. I have been asked many times if we become emotionally cold in order to deal with the sadness inherent in our profession. It could not be further from the truth. Time and experience teach us of the strengths and vulnerabilities of humans, that the decisions we make can have lifelong effects on our patients and on ourselves. Sometimes it is easier to operate than not to operate, even when we know that it will not benefit our patients, because often the disease holds all the cards.

What I do know is that the relationship between surgeon and patient is a special one. There is no other profession in which a perfect stranger trusts you with their life after an hour, maybe two. Our patients sign a piece of paper allowing us to enter their bodies, entrusting that while they are unconscious they will be treated with the utmost care, and that we will do our very best for them. In particular, they trust that we will not harm them. This agreement, in all words said and unsaid, demands empathy from the surgeon and not a cold heart. For our patients, empathy always matters.

However, as I would come to learn, this empathy is far easier with a patient than with a sick family member. What happens when there is no agreement and it is just blood that assumes this? The relationship between a sick family member and you as a carer is much less clear, and much more difficult. Under many medical council regulations across the world, including in New Zealand, it is deemed inappropriate to treat family. But, while we do not treat our families directly, there is often an expectation that we will be heavily involved in the decisions or directions for their care, and this affects our freedom to grieve as a child, as a husband or wife, as a family member. Moreover, because we are human, these situations are always coloured by the past, by indiscretions and injustices, by the fact that we are family.

* * *

A month after the start of my first consultancy year, I had a call from my mother. She had not opened her bowels for over a week. As a general surgeon, my instant reaction was alarm. 'That is not good, Mum. I am not happy about that at all,' I told her. 'Are you farting?' Farting is so very important to general surgeons, as it demonstrates gas can exit from the bowels and therefore passage is patent. When one develops a bowel obstruction, farting stops.

'Yes,' she replied. 'I am fine. I am drinking green tea and I think I can feel things moving.'

'Okay, but if you haven't moved anything by the end of the week, you need to come over,' I instructed.

I knew she would not want to. My father had returned to Samoa by this time, and required a degree of supervision, as he was on anti-epileptic medication, could no longer drive and had lost his social life. Since he essentially had a significant brain injury, he was increasingly unreasonable and perseverant. Every bad behaviour he'd had in his personality profile before his illness was augmented. He was quick to anger and totally irrational. Furthermore, the debt he had amassed was not going to be payable by either of my parents in their lifetimes.

My mother was working overtime to keep everything afloat. By that, I mean that she was working to cover my father's multiple monthly repayments to multiple banks. 'You need to let everything fall, Mum,' I kept pestering her. 'You cannot keep working just to pay this off, and nor can your children.' (I was referring to my sister, who had decided to stay with my mother and help her with the business.) 'Let him declare bankruptcy, or have him declared incompetent even!'

I felt desperate for my mother and my sister, and it was tearing our relationship apart. I could not deal with the same complaints every time we spoke on the phone, and she was almost certainly tired of me telling her to leave everything behind her. She could not. She had a loyalty – probably not to her husband, but to her children – and was committed to trying to keep their home of over 30 years.

I called her the following week to ask if things were better. 'Yes, I am fine,' she said. 'Everything is good now.' Our conversations were getting shorter. She knew I did not want to hear what was happening, but she could not speak of anything else because her life was consuming her.

* * *

About six months passed before my sister called. 'Mum is not well. She has been having severe abdominal pain, and today she has been really bad.'

'Shit.' I sighed. 'Get her on the plane, please.'

I already knew what it was going to be. I had seen this sort of story unfold often enough to know what a scan of her abdomen would show – but I still hoped it could be benign.

Within days of her arrival, she had a CT colonography of her bowel. This is a virtual colonoscopy, a study we could get access to quickly. I received a call from the radiologist later that evening confirming her diagnosis: my mother had a very large cancer on the left side of her colon, wrapping circumferentially around the bowel and causing a near-obstruction, with spread outside the colon. It was well advanced. Not truly metastatic, but not good.

'Was that the radiologist?' my mother asked as soon as I put the phone down.

'Yes,' I said honestly, wishing that I could have a bit more time to myself to think. We had just finished pulling life together around one unwell parent. Now we were going to embark on another journey for my mother. We were sitting in the living room, and the sofa bed that my son had been demoted to was pulled out and ready for him. 'You have a bowel cancer, Mum,' I said. How weird to say it to your own parent. With a patient, it sounded better practised. I almost did not know how to say it emotionally, because I had said it over and over so many times before.

'Is it bad?' she asked. This is a normal reaction.

'It is big,' I told her. 'It can be removed with surgery, but you will definitely need chemotherapy.'

She cried, and I put my arm around her. I reassured her, but I felt like it was empty. We sat on the couch but we had already fallen deep into our thoughts. Would it have been this bad if she had got on the plane earlier? What would happen with the repayments in Samoa? How could we make space here for her to stay?

My mother started moving along the pathway that I knew like the back of my hand: more scans, a colonoscopy, biopsies, blood tests, anaesthetists, surgery. I had her operated on by the best surgeon I knew, one who would treat her the way she was to me: my mother. The only person who would do this was my mentor. It remains one of my regrets that I did not go into theatre with her to see her off to sleep that day. Instead, I went to clinic.

The scan had underestimated the extent of my mother's disease, as it is known to do. She had cancer outside the colon and involving multiple lymph nodes. Nonetheless, she had an extensive resection of all the local disease and the palpable nodes that ran up alongside the major vessel in her abdomen – but, when I saw on her final histology that all those nodes were positive, I knew she was in a fight for her life.

We decided she needed to live with me, but my son and I were moving in a few months to a new city so I could take up another job. She would have to come with us.

* * *

While my mother was having her colon cancer treated, I was operating on others with colon cancer. Mr C came into hospital complaining of pelvic pain, abdominal distension and a change in bowel habit. He had been fit and well up until the few weeks before his symptoms started. He was a lively man, 64 years of age, with no other medical problems. He wore his own clothes in hospital – always a sign – and he was immaculate even though he was unwell.

A CT scan of his abdomen revealed a very large obstructing cancer in the left part of his colon, which had dropped down low into the pelvis and grown into the top part of his rectum. Fortunately, despite the size of the colonic cancer, there was no evidence of cancer anywhere else. Cancer is a funny beast like that. Sometimes we locate a small malignancy that has spread to the liver and lungs; at other times, we see very large cancers, such as the one Mr C had, but all the distant organs remain pristine. (Or we see cases like my mother's, where the cancer is both large and has already spread extensively through the nodes.) Nevertheless, most tumours obey the rules, and in general, size gives us information for staging and prognosis.

Mr C's cancer was causing an obstruction and he needed surgery quickly. Specifically, he needed a large part of his left colon and his rectum removed. First, he required a resection of the lower end of his colon (called the sigmoid colon), because this was where the primary cancer had flourished. He also required resection of his rectum to the top of the anal canal, because the tumour had grown into the rectum itself.

Lymph nodes travel along the arteries that supply the colon, and the arterial supply of the colon is segmented by location: right, middle and left. When we are performing a cancer resection of the colon, it is imperative to remove the draining lymph nodes, and thus the arteries along which they travel. Hence, the entire section of colon supplied by the artery also needs to be removed so that fresh, healthy ends can be re-joined. This join is called an anastomosis. To heal, an anastomosis requires good blood supply, otherwise it will break down and faeces will leak freely into the abdominal cavity.

This is why, for even a small cancer in the right side of the colon, we have to take the right colonic artery to clear all the lymph nodes, which might harbour tiny cancer cells from the primary lesion. Also, as the blood supply to the right colon has been sacrificed, it is necessary to take the right colon so that only healthy bowel is left behind. Patients always wonder why we have to remove an amount of colon disproportionately larger than a tiny cancer, so I was well familiar with quickly drawing the colon and its blood vessels over and over again in an afternoon clinic.

When we re-join bowel to the top of the anal canal, the risk of an anastomotic leak is in the region of 10 per cent. This means that one out of every ten people who has this operation will have an anastomotic breakdown, with faeces leaking into their pelvis. This causes them to become critically unwell and they will most likely require second surgery and intensive care. For this reason, when we perform these high-risk anastomoses so low in the pelvis, we bring out a defunctioning stoma – it is temporary and allows the effluent of stool to bypass the fresh anastomosis, which lies further downstream. It does not reduce the risk of an anastomotic leak, but because stools will not be traversing the anastomosis it reduces the risk of sepsis and reoperation.

Needless to say, Mr C also needed a stoma. Of course, there are more risks than an anastomotic leak alone. There is also the risk of inadvertent injury to adjacent bowel or solid organs, the risk of clots in the legs or the clot moving to the lungs (pulmonary embolus), and the risks related to anaesthesia. And, given the extent of pelvic surgery that Mr C required, the risk of impotence was significant – probably in the order of about 30 per cent.

He was prepared for surgery within 24 hours, consented and had a stoma site marked on his abdominal wall by the stoma nurse. The surgery itself was challenging. A large cancer sitting in a narrow male pelvis always makes us work a little harder. All the necessary structures were identified – the ureter, the pelvic vessels, the plexus of nerves responsible for erection and ejaculation – and the large cancer was removed en bloc with the sigmoid colon, the rectum, and all the lymph nodes and the fatty tissue in which they lay. The left colon around the spleen was freed from its attachments, and brought down on its blood supply into the pelvis. The anastomosis was fashioned routinely, then a stoma was brought out on the right side.

Mr C made a stellar recovery. His final pathology told us he would have a small benefit from chemotherapy on the basis of the tumour's size, and the fact that it had breached the colonic wall from which it originated and had also invaded the rectum. Fortunately, the 26 lymph nodes that were removed were all clear. After a week in hospital, Mr C was discharged.

When he came in to the clinic for his six-week follow-up, he informed us that he did not want chemotherapy and begged for his stoma to be reversed. It turned out that he had met a new young lover and wanted to have sexual relations with her – without the stoma bag and the toxicity of chemotherapy. After ensuring he understood very clearly all his options, I closed the stoma for him. The operation went swimmingly well, and he sent me vintage bottles of champagne for his sex life and the erection that he was still able to achieve.

* * *

By my thirty-fifth year, I had been a student in the art of surgery for a decade, and a fully qualified surgeon for two of those years. I was privileged to have been part of many happy stories, and equally privileged to have been part of many sad ones.

We are truly in the industry of people, and this was one of the things I loved most about general surgery. I was not invited into my patients' lives. Often, I was there when their lives took a turn for the unimaginable. Many of us never imagine that one day we will be diagnosed with a terminal illness or told that a loved one is fighting for their life. It is at these moments that the general surgeon, much like a wrecking ball, swings into the picture. For this reason, the reward can be maximal. When people present with life-threatening illness or trauma, you can save a life. But general surgery never lets you forget that, with great heights, a fall can come.

What a strange job it is that when I recall that year – my thirty-fifth – it is deaths on the operating table and deaths off it that come to mind. By this time, I had been subject to a Health and Disciplinary Commission (HDC) inquiry not once but twice. Is 35 too young for that? I know that particular anxiety when a thick brown envelope arrives with that legal look about it and it is addressed to you. You receive it once and you never forget the weight of it. Inside, there will be a letter bulldog-clipped to a patient's thick medical record asking you for a witness statement or telling you that the HDC is investigating whether your actions might have contributed directly to mortality. Was the patient's death avoidable? It's a fair enough question.

Did I ever go into medicine or surgery knowing or even contemplating that one day I might be held responsible for a death? Does any one of us? The simple answer is no. My goal was always to prevent it. My goal *is* to prevent it. My goal is to make people better and get them back to normal. We spend at least ten years of our lives training to be surgeons. We spend days and nights – 24 hours, 72 hours, weekends, loved ones' birthdays, children's swimming lessons and Saturday-morning sports matches – in this apprenticeship. We sacrifice just about everything. But we are human. We are not perfect. Despite these endless nights and days, the thousands of operative cases, we make mistakes. And the worst of these outcomes – *death* – frequent as it may be around us as surgeons, is always difficult. So, what do I say to my friends and family when they ask how we cope with the sadness? You have no idea, but how can I explain it to you? Surgery is an insular world.

My non-medical friends also in their thirties – okay, you got me, I had very few because my job made it difficult to maintain friends off the roster – had never contemplated the magnitude of being blamed for a death. And a handful of times, as I put my clothes back on in the middle of the night to return to the hospital, I envied them. Did they keep jeans, socks, underwear and a sweater at the foot of the bed so as not to waste time if they were called back to work in the middle of the night? Anyone in surgery knows the solitude of driving back to the hospital at 3 a.m. The Devil's hour, my father used to call it. It is an hour when the only occupants of the street are rubbish bins waiting for collection the next morning. How many times have I driven past such rubbish bins wondering if their owners are warm and happy in their beds?

It was a 2 a.m. awakening for one woman who had been on the medical ward, rehabilitating after an operation, in a peripheral hospital a two-hour ambulance drive away. Earlier that evening, she had deteriorated rapidly, and by the time she got to us and was brought to theatre, she was barely responsive because of overwhelming sepsis and shock.

I felt myself going into shock also – but, rather than the medical shock and organ shutdown of my patient, mine was the shock born of a sudden and unexpected event in the middle of the night. I was already exhausted after a long day of operating. My legs ached, and my feet were swollen. I contemplated putting on my thigh-high compression stockings, but at that hour it was too much of an effort. Those things are difficult enough to get on at 8 a.m. As I walked past the mirror on my way out of the theatre bathroom, I contemplated putting on make-up – I looked so sallow – but instead chose the scrub hat and mask that could hide a number of sins.

When I saw the patient's shape underneath her hospital gown while the anaesthetist was busy putting her to sleep, tears of distress and fatigue stung my eyes. She was morbidly obese, which always makes a surgeon's heart sink, particularly in the middle of the night. I would need a very good assistant to help me, and I would need the largest surgical retractors to hold open a very big wound. This operation was going to be a physical challenge. My neck and shoulders ached in anticipation of what lay ahead.

She had earnt herself an incision up and down her abdomen, from the bottom of her ribcage to the top of her pubic bone. An abdominal catastrophe requires no less. In this case, the catastrophe was inadvertent injury to her bowel during a gynaecological operation three days prior. Faeces had been leaking out of a hole in her colon, and every corner of her abdominal cavity was filled with liquid brown. No wonder she was so sick.

We excised the section of bowel that had been damaged and, with much difficulty due to its size, brought a stoma out to the abdominal wall. That was followed by a ten-litre warm saline wash to rid her abdominal cavity of every morsel of faecal material. The smell of faeces filled our nostrils as the warm wash spilt over our legs and shoes. I asked for her to be tilted away from me, so that I was not so inundated by it. I could already feel that the wash had found its way over the top of my gloves and through my gown, soaking my arms. It is never a welcome warmth, and I did not want to be soaked any further as I'd only brought one pair of knickers to work that night. At 3 a.m., this thought was hilarious.

I was still elbow-deep in her abdomen when the on-call registrar arrived in theatre to inform us there was another emergency. Sometimes, the messenger can bear the brunt of disbelief. I glared at this junior registrar while he gave me a summary of the next patient, and I yearned to find a hole in his story. It is only emergencies that we are allowed to operate on overnight. This makes sense: no one is at their best in the wee hours, plus staffing is minimal. So, unless it is life or limb, it must wait until the morning. It is safer for the patient, and for us. But waiting until sunrise had not been possible for the woman who was about to be wheeled out of theatre with a new stoma, and nor was it an option for the woman who the registrar was telling me about.

She was in her eighties, and had been brought in unresponsive by the ambulance. An assessment in the emergency department confirmed that she had a bowel perforation, probably caused by a stomach ulcer. She needed an operation to save her life. The problem was, however, that the 30-day mortality for an octogenarian presenting with an abdominal catastrophe that requires emergency surgery is around 25 per cent. This means that, within 30 days, one in four people over 80 who undergo emergency abdominal surgery will die. Of course, this has to be weighed against a 100 per cent risk of dying without surgery. But there is so much more to the former – the risk of a stroke or heart attack, the risk of death during surgery, the risk of lung failure, the risk of being dependent on a ventilator after surgery, the risk that we need to go back to theatre within 24 hours. And, if the patient gets through it all, there's also the risk of not returning to the same level of function with which they came into the hospital. Therefore, after establishing that this woman needed an operation, I also had to establish what her normal level of functionality was – whether she had family, and whether operating would be in accordance with her wishes. It is a lot to consider when time is of the essence, and it's horrible pressure to place on a patient and their family at a desperate time.

'Don't operate on someone who will die tomorrow,' a senior colleague once told me. But how do you know? It was established that, in fact, this woman was as sharp as a razor blade. She lived at home completely independently, and had no medical problems – a brilliant medical résumé for an 80-year-old woman. After ascertaining that she would have wanted life-saving surgery, and that her family did not want anything less, I prepared them for the worst. I would do my best, I informed them, but she had a big fight ahead of her.

At some time after 4 a.m., she was transferred to the operating table, where we patched up her stomach ulcer. And, while I was still in the operating theatre with her, I learnt that a 34-year-old man was being moved into the emergency department by ambulance staff. His car had been hit side-on by another car travelling at high speed, and a trauma call had gone out for him after the emergency staff were notified of his impending arrival. When paramedics attend a scene and find serious injuries, they alert triage in the nearest (or most suitable) emergency department, and a trauma call is generated to the hospital's trauma team, which usually includes on-call doctors from the emergency department, general surgery and intensive care. Thereafter, other specialties are called in as required.

The trauma team descended on the resuscitation bay and waited to receive him. His upper body had taken most of the impact: both his collarbones were clearly broken, and it was easy to appreciate his rib fractures also. A systematic assessment of his airway, breathing and circulation took place and then, as is routine in such a high-risk mechanism of injury, he had a scan of his entire body to elucidate the severity of his injuries, and to make sure there was no other occult injury. He had sustained multiple injuries: five left rib fractures, fractures of both collarbones, a complex and unstable pelvic fracture, a left pneumothorax (popped lung) and a splenic laceration.

A tube was placed into his chest to drain the air and allow the lung to expand again and seal. His collarbone and rib fractures would be managed with generous pain relief. His unstable pelvis required a binder. The laceration to his spleen was not actively bleeding, and therefore did not require an intervention at that moment, but it did require careful observation. Splenic lacerations carry a risk of bleeding, and that risk rises with the severity of the laceration. For each organ injury, he had a different set of specialists who knew more about that particular part of the body than anyone else: a thoracic surgery team for his lung, an orthopaedic surgery team for his collarbones and pelvis, and a general surgical team for his spleen. He was admitted to the intensive care unit overnight, as it was the best place for the one-on-one nursing and close observation he required.

This all unfolded while I was still operating on the woman in her eighties, but I had been kept well informed by the junior registrar as the man's story progressed. It was one of those nights when I felt akin to a soldier among the dead and dying. The night in theatre had left me drained, so once I had news that the young man was stable in the intensive care unit I grabbed a few hours of sleep then went and met him for the first time. He was more effusive than I would have expected given his injuries. Comfortable, sitting upright in bed, his only concern was when he might be able to get back to his cage-fighting (martial arts).

I studied his scan, I checked his blood tests, I remarked on how stable his observations had been, then I ordered strict bedrest, which is routine for a laceration to the spleen. I did not want him jumping out of bed and causing further disruption and trauma. 'It will be a minimum of six weeks before you can get back to your cage-fighting,' I told him. He will be fine, I thought confidently.

* * *

I returned home to spend the weekend with my mother. We were having a coffee the next morning when my phone rang.

'The man who was in the traffic accident was found dead in his bed this morning. His observations had been perfect all night, but his nurse found him dead at 8 a.m. Sorry.'

My ears were ringing, and my heart was racing. I was in disbelief. What had I missed? I felt sick. I was also terrified. Had I overlooked something important that had ultimately led to his demise?

'What's wrong?' my mother asked, sensing my distress.

'Nothing,' I replied abruptly.

My appetite for breakfast and time with others had crashed to zero, but my mother knew her daughter well. She did not push.

Within another 24 hours, both ladies who had kept me up all night were also dead, and I was under investigation in relation to the man. Evidently, both doing and *not* doing can cause harm.

Weeks of sleepless nights ensued. All I could see when I closed my eyes was the man's face. A 34-year-old should not be found dead in his hospital bed. What had I done wrong? How could his death have been prevented? I felt haunted. I spent weeks calling colleagues to ask whether they would have done anything differently.

First, do no harm. Easier said than done.

6.

Who teaches death and dying?

On a normal evening on call, with an eager fourth-year medical student in tow, my registrar stumbled on a great teaching case. The registrar was overcome with enthusiasm, and the medical student was bright with anticipation.

A woman had died on the ward, and the registrar on duty thought it would be fantastic to teach our student how to certify a death. The registrar herself had not learnt how to do this until she was nearly a full-fledged doctor – obviously a couple of years too late in her own mind. For most of us, declaring a death remains a harrowing experience and, not infrequently, the first time you are asked to do so is in the middle of the night in your first month as a doctor. It can be an unpleasant experience, and the memory fills me with anxiety even now.

The ward is never so quiet as when you must certify a death in the dead of night. The lights are usually off so that all the other patients can sleep, except for the single dim light that beckons you into the room of the recently deceased. In most cases, it is very important that you do *not* go into the room immediately after the ward nurse calls you to certify a death in the middle of the night. (The obvious exception to this is when the death is completely unexpected, in which case you should put on your running shoes.) Declaring someone dead requires the following: absence of heart sounds for one minute, absence of a pulse for one minute, absence of breathing for one minute and unreactive pupils. You don't want to attempt the certification too early for fear of hearing a runaway breath or heart sound, as this can irrevocably shake the very thin foundation of confidence you have as a junior doctor. In addition to that, the family are also often there, as you would expect, and this can make the certification very awkward if you have even an ounce of uncertainty.

Such important pearls of wisdom are imparted from one doctor to another, so the registrar rightly thought that she was bestowing invaluable knowledge upon the soon-to-be junior doctor. She had not considered that it would be traumatic for a student at the tender age of 21 to be confronted with declaring her first death on the ward. And of course, to the registrar's surprise, as soon as they entered the cubicle of the deceased, the student turned pale, asked quickly to be excused and fled.

Why didn't we consider that seeing and touching a dead body might shock a young medical student? This 21-year-old medical student would have to face things that her lawyer and accountant peers would never encounter. How do we prepare medical students to see and accept death? When did we, as doctors, start to accept it?

The truth is that death and dying are difficult for us to deal with at all moments of our careers. For surgeons, the confrontation of death is acute. 'What we do is fucked up,' a friend and colleague said in passing one day. I knew he was right – I had been contemplating death and dying, and how we are not always equipped to deal with it – but what he said caught me off guard because, as colleagues, we rarely speak of how death affects us. 'I finally understand how the enemy of good is better,' he said, before going on to recount an oesophagectomy he'd done in a minimally invasive fashion (laparoscopically). After completing the chest part of the operation, he decided at the last minute to open one last attachment for good measure – but this resulted in blood pouring into the chest and the operative field. He had gone into the major blood vessel leaving the heart.

We are trained for events like this. It is a common exam scenario: you are doing a splenectomy (removing the spleen) when the abdomen fills with blood. How do you approach this? I could recite the answer in my sleep. *Put pressure on it. Alert your anaesthetist and let them catch up. Make sure the lights are in place and you can see well. Get your retractors ready and put them in place. Tell the theatre nurses to set up two suctions. Get lots of packs ready.* But actually putting a hole in the aorta and having your operating field fill with blood puts the fear of God into you.

Systematically, my friend went through the checklist: he told the anaesthetist and the team what had happened, he told them what he needed, he waited until everyone was ready, he took a deep breath to steady himself, and he fixed the hole.

He was obviously still aware of what could have happened that day as he told me this story. Afterwards, he said, he had gone home, mentioned that it was a tough day at work, and nothing more. He explained how his ex-girlfriend had been unhappy with him because he did not – or could not – share. But how can you explain to someone other than a surgeon that your patient could have died on the operating table, and now you have lead in your chest and you feel sick to your stomach and can't sleep?

* * *

Pelvic surgery can be tough. I have seen it bring consultants to their knees – literally – when bleeding from the pelvis could not be stopped.

The only time I ever felt sick during surgery was in the middle of a pelvic operation. The man was having an open radical prostatectomy, because he had prostate cancer and required removal of his entire prostate. At that time, this was done in an open fashion as a routine, as opposed to laparoscopically or robotically, as we now see more commonly. Males have a narrower pelvis than females, who bear children and therefore have a wider inlet, and access can be difficult. Such was the case for this man, who also had a very large prostate. A discordant relationship – narrow pelvis with large prostate – makes things even more difficult. He bled a lot, and I recall the pelvis filling with blood quicker than we could control it. The sweet, warm smell penetrated my mask and a wave of nausea washed over me, as I had been standing there for hours in an uncomfortable position, sweating because of the lights directly overhead. However, I dutifully held the retractors and the suction, and bore the brunt of the abuse from the consultant. He wasn't able to see where the blood was coming from, and neither my suction nor my retraction was helping him. Finally, after a few units of blood and surgical adjuncts for haemostasis, the field was dry and there was no more bleeding. We closed the patient up and moved him off the table.

I glanced over at the surgeon. He had unscrubbed and walked to the other side of the theatre, where he was now sitting with his head in his hands, rocking back and forth on the chair. I was a little stunned as I watched him. He was obviously stunned too. It made me realise how close to the edge surgeons are. One cannot imagine how it feels to be so close to losing a patient.

I was operating one day when the nurses were complaining about another surgeon and his unacceptable behaviour. He did high-risk surgery, where catastrophic bleeding could occur, and was known to throw instruments when stressed. I did not condone this behaviour – however, having worked with him, I also knew he thanked everyone individually at the end of each case, and if I ever needed his help as a trainee surgeon he was there without hesitation. I am not sure if it is logical that good behaviour cancels bad, but he was a great surgeon, and I always believed that those who complained could not possibly understand what it was like to have a patient's life in their hands. Meanwhile, the surgeon I was with that day was far from demonstrative and was clearly withdrawing, and I felt helpless. Sometimes, we just have to start with the little things. 'Let me consent the next patient and get him ready, then I'll grab you a coffee and let's meet in the tearoom,' I said in as light a voice as possible.

* * *

A senior registrar sat next to me as we were waiting in theatre for a procedure to start. (We spend a lot of time in theatre waiting for procedures to start.) He'd had a tough couple of weeks, and it had all begun with an evening on call and a sick man in the emergency department.

The man was 30 years old and had presented unwell with a fever, low blood pressure and a rapid heart rate. He was morbidly obese, weighing 160 kilograms, and unsurprisingly diabetic, which is an expected co-occurrence. In patients with obesity, the body becomes immune to circulating insulin, and the result is that blood sugar rages out of control as it escapes the hypoglycaemic effect of insulin. The high blood sugars impact the ability of the body's white blood cells to fight infection, making the person very susceptible to life-threatening infection — and, in this man's case, from his soft tissue and fat.

Earlier that afternoon, a family member had found him unrousable and called the ambulance. Apparently, he had complained during the week of anal pain and had experienced increasing difficulty sitting for any length of time. Examination of this region was difficult given his size, but it was clear that he had a severe and extensive infection in his buttocks, which had more than likely started as a result of a blocked gland in his anal canal. His skin was blistered, and his scrotum was dark grey. Based on his vitals, the examination and his blood tests, he had what we call necrotising fasciitis. Known in lay terms as the flesh-eating disease, this is a severe infection of fat and soft tissue with a fatality rate that approaches 80 per cent. This man was in trouble.

He was taken to theatre for emergency surgery, which would not be an easy task with a patient weighing 160 kilograms. From the start, he was unstable, his blood pressure and heart rate plummeting at induction of anaesthesia.

Theatres are always full of people in critical cases such as this, and there is a nervous energy. The anaesthetic team are always at the top end of the table, and often in these critically unwell patients, or when an airway has the potential to be difficult, there will be two anaesthetists. There is also the anaesthetic technician, who assists with the intubation and lines (the plastic tubes inserted into veins to infuse anaesthetic, antibiotics, pain relief and, as in this case, blood pressure support). The anaesthetists and the technician stood at the head of the table with the defibrillator as the man floated towards cardiac arrest.

He needed large bore lines and one was placed in his neck with direct access to his heart. He also needed a line in his artery to measure his blood pressure accurately. Trying to take a blood pressure reading from a standard cuff was impossible given his size. All this takes time, and rightly so, because patients can crash at induction of anaesthesia if they are very unwell. And, while the anaesthetists are busy ensuring a critical patient can stably enter anaesthesia, the surgeons are waiting at the bottom of the table predictably eager to get started. Maybe even impatiently pacing or tapping a foot combined with frequent glances at the clock. The nurses are in and out of the theatre to make sure the surgeons have the equipment they need. The scrub nurse can be seen counting her instruments, while another nurse circulates in theatre. The count is repeated at the end of the case to make sure nothing is left behind in a body cavity.

The air on this day was electric. Surgery for these cases is, for want of a better word, gruesome. The tissue is essentially dead, and you have to cut with a scalpel until you get to tissue that bleeds. The patient was on his back with his heavy legs in stirrups, and once the anaesthetists gave us the nod the registrar began removing kilos of dead tissue with a blade – all the tissue over the man's inner thighs, perineum, anterior abdominal wall and testicles was surgically removed. It is not elegant surgery, nor is it kind, but it is lifesaving.

The man's buttocks were also dead, but they were inaccessible with him on his back. So, in order to access his posterior, this 160-kilogram man had to be turned over on to his stomach by eight members of staff. And it was in this position that his heart stopped. Disaster. He needed to be turned back over again immediately.

The emergency bell was pressed. In theatre, this brings a mass of people straightaway. Everyone who was present helped to turn him once again, and CPR was commenced. Several rounds of CPR ensued before the man was declared dead. A 30-year-old dead on the table. It was not right. The registrar, and no doubt everyone involved, was clearly shaken.

* * *

Now, just under two weeks later, this registrar and I were waiting in theatre for another critical patient. We had not yet finished our conversation when we were called to open the patient, who had been admitted with bleeding from somewhere in his gut. The bleeding was brisk, and he was unstable, so he required intensive care immediately.

'You operated on him two years ago,' my admitting registrar said to me.

'What?' I replied in alarm. It is always a moment of dread when you encounter a patient you have operated on before. Your immediate thought is, What did I do wrong? In this case, it turned out that I had operated on the man's simple groin hernia, which had no relation to his current predicament.

A scan had demonstrated that the bleeding was probably coming from somewhere in his stomach, but more importantly he had spots in his liver, suggesting he had metastatic cancer. This always changes our treatment pathway. Making a big incision in someone's abdomen is an easy task, however – and as I always say to my patients – everything we do has a risk. We knew only that he had metastatic cancer, not whether it was a cancer that would respond well to chemotherapy, or what this cancer meant for his life expectancy. We wanted to treat him in a way that would allow him to recover quickly. If he had only three months left to live, then at least he would not have to spend most of his time recovering from a big operation. These are the things we must weigh up.

Initially, we never planned to open him at all. Instead, we had been hoping to control the bleeding with a minimally invasive procedure through a blood vessel in his groin. Unfortunately, as soon as he was anaesthetised his blood pressure plummeted, so we had no choice but to open him and control the bleeding quickly with a maximally invasive procedure. I could hear the stress in the registrar's voice as he requested instruments and asked for the lights to be repositioned, and for silence so that he could communicate with the anaesthetist. His stress manifested in the pitch and tone of his voice, and his increasingly short temper. He shouted unnecessarily at the scrub nurse, and his movements were inefficient.

It occurred to me that he was traumatised because of his last couple of weeks, and it made me wonder how any of us got through to the other end of training in some semblance of normal. I know that most of us simply bear the trauma and continue. Personally, I have felt devastated by the loss of every single patient, but you keep going; the job is busy, and every day you count on the fact that you will feel better with time. No one tells you there is any other way to do it. When a colleague in another hospital saw a junior registrar traumatised after a critical event in theatre, she tried to set up a support network for any member of staff – junior or senior – who might require a friendly ear or a debrief. Imagine her surprise when she was told by two of the most senior members of the department that such a group was not required. Apparently, you should just get on with things.

In the end, the man we'd had to open never woke up. His life support was turned off in intensive care.

The sadness hits like a kick in the guts.

* * *

One of my clearest memories as a medical student is spending a night in the delivery suite. Just months away from graduating from medical school, I was assigned to a night shift with the obstetric registrar on call.

It was after midnight, and I was stealing sleep in the tearoom in a moment of stillness. But it was just a moment. I was startled awake by the registrar, who asked me to follow him. A woman had been in labour throughout the afternoon, and there was now foetal distress. He handed me the cardiotocograph, which monitors foetal heart rate and uterine contractions, and explained that what we were seeing were decelerations and a scalp pH that was grossly abnormal. The decelerations meant that the foetal heart rate was decreasing, and the scalp pH confirmed that the baby was lacking oxygen and was in grave trouble.

The exhausted mother was wheeled rapidly down the corridor for an emergency caesarean section. The anaesthetic and obstetric consultants had been called, and they were rushing in. Meanwhile, the mother, who had a good epidural in place was ready for an incision.

I stood opposite the registrar, waiting for him to begin, and I will never forget his hands. They shook violently, the blade in his right hand. He was terrified, and I could hear him hyperventilating through his mask. This was the first time I had met him, so I did not know how many times he had done this, but it seemed as though the weight of the operating theatre was on him. The obstetric consultant entered the room. 'Why the fuck haven't you started?' he screamed.

The theatre was full and everyone knew the situation was bad. The mother, who was awake at the head of the table, with her husband beside her, was being 'shielded' by one of the nurses. This is normal. There is always someone at the head of the table, explaining what is happening, doing their best to reassure the mother, telling her that the noises and the number of people in theatre is to be expected. I am unsure if this mother registered that it was not good; undoubtedly she finally did when the obstetrician made his presence known. The paediatricians and the neonatal intensivists were waiting, all hoping for the best. As the registrar made the first incision, his chest heaved underneath his theatre gown, his breathing audible. I held the edges of the wound open with the retractors he handed me, and kept following him until he went through the muscular wall that had housed a foetus for nine months. The obstetric consultant, who had scrubbed in at this point, seized the position as primary surgeon and I was moved down the table.

The baby was blue when we finally retrieved it from the open uterus. It did not breathe spontaneously and could not be resuscitated.

I have no words to describe the devastation in the theatre that night. My eyes stung with tears as we closed.

The registrar left medicine shortly after that event. I have no idea what happened to him. I am not sure anyone asked.

* * *

My first encounter with death as a young doctor had been in my first six weeks as a new graduate. It was expected: she was in her eighties and had been unwell on the ward with a pneumonia. She had deteriorated in the afternoon and, knowing that I was going to be on call, I went in to see her. She was delirious, talking of things that I could not see. It was sad to see that she was alone, without any family or loved ones by her side. She died three hours later, and the nurses called me so that I could certify the death and start the paperwork.

I was anxious to do this before the sun went down, so I went back up to the ward within an hour of the call. She was not yet cold, but she was so still. Everything in her cubicle was still, as if not even air was moving through it. I caught my own breath, quickly went through the necessary checks and left.

The next death, and I will never forget it, was a two-year-old girl who had a severe developmental delay. She had been critically unwell on the paediatric ward and was deteriorating rapidly. The paediatric surgeon decided we needed to look inside her abdomen, so she came to theatre. She was so sick. She died on the table.

I was assisting, and the surgeon left me to close her up so that her parents could hold her. I cried as I sutured her up, and as I left to see the other patients waiting to be assessed in the emergency department I walked past the nurses. They were crying in the scrub bay.

* * *

Sometimes, it is our patients' bravery that really strikes us. They can be fit and well when they walk into hospital, and walk out with a life expectancy measured in weeks. These patients must take in this information while lying in a hospital bed, then take stock of what they have and immediately begin to make arrangements for a world without them in six to eight weeks' time.

Mr W, a man in his seventies without a single medical problem, had been referred by his general practitioner. He was jaundiced, and a blood test demonstrated a bilirubin level over 300. Bilirubin is produced in the liver, and stored in the gallbladder, a small organ sheltered under the liver's free edge. It is usually excreted from the liver into the small bowel through a tube called the bile duct.

When I looked at Mr W, there was no doubt his bilirubin was grossly abnormal: he was a putrid shade of green, a colour that is extremely telling and means certain death within weeks. Someone who presents this colour, without pain or fever, almost certainly has cancer. He had other classic symptoms and signs that go along with this degree of jaundice, too – he was a little confused, his arms and torso showed scratch marks (which confirmed the itch that bilirubin build-up portends), his urine was very dark and his stools were pale. He was thin, and we could feel his gallbladder by pressing gently underneath his right ribcage. There is a name for this: Courvoisier's sign. So named after the man who first described this finding: Monsieur Courvoisier.

Medicine has many disorders named after the first man, or (rarely) woman, who decided to put their name to the condition. Unfortunately, Courvoisier's sign is not good. A CT scan of Mr W's body confirmed this. He did indeed have cancer. It had likely originated in his bile duct, and his liver was full of it.

There was nothing we could do. Nothing even to relieve the jaundice to make him feel better. Two weeks earlier, he had been completely well. Fit and active, playing an 18-hole round of golf with friends, and now we were telling him that he was dying, that it would be within weeks, and that he could decide if he wished to die at home or in the hospice.

Within another two weeks, he died, surrounded by his wife and family and friends.

If you are in medicine, you know this is a good way to go. Enough time to say goodbye, but not long enough to suffer.

* * *

I was rostered on for two weeks of general surgical call, clinics and operating in the regions. Mr O was admitted during one of these weeks, with profuse vomiting and back pain. He was 68 years old, and until two months prior had been completely fit and well, lived at home with his wife and owned a business. Then he had been diagnosed with pancreatic cancer, and it had been deemed inoperable because it was wrapped around important vessels and could not be peeled off them safely, and nor could the vessels be resected and reconstructed.

On arrival at the emergency department, Mr O was given a CT scan, and I was subsequently called. He had quite marked progression of his pancreatic cancer. It was much larger, and had involved yet another important vessel. This dramatic increase in size explained his back pain, for which he required large amounts of morphine. The scan also demonstrated that the cancer was compressing the duodenum (the first part of the small intestine), which normally forms a C-shape around the pancreas in health and was therefore vulnerable to compression from a pancreatic head mass. The duodenum was obstructed, and Mr O's stomach was full of fluid. This explained the vomiting. He had been waiting to get to chemotherapy, which in the absence of surgery was his only option for more time. The chemotherapy, however, would never cure him.

'In my experience, he should be put in the hospice and palliated,' the young doctor had said to me after he had finished making his referral by phone.

'What experience would that be?' I had replied, probably too sharply. Palliative care is a hugely important specialty in end-of-life care. For us specifically as surgeons, it means that treatment is withdrawn, and that the focus shifts to managing debilitating symptoms, such as pain and nausea, before death (whenever that might be).

Despite the progression of the cancer, Mr O did not have evidence at that moment of gross distant disease, and he had previously been fit and well. I knew that, even if we were to put him in the hospice and palliate him, it would not be quick. His cause of death would have to be starvation. A horrible way to go.

When I spoke to Mr O and his wife, I explained that the cancer appeared to have grown significantly, in a short space of time. 'But our immediate problem is the obstruction,' I said. 'You have three options. One, we can put a stent – a metal tube – into the duodenum to hold the passage open, but often with massive external compression the stent will fail quite quickly, and you will re-obstruct. Two, we can perform an open operation to bring a loop of small bowel up to the stomach to join them, so that the stomach drains freely into the small bowel and bypasses the duodenum completely, but there is risk with an open operation. Or three, we can do nothing. We can admit you to the hospice, where they will keep you comfortable, but there is no reason that you will die imminently. In the end, you will die of starvation.'

They quickly ruled out options one and three, and we spoke more about option two. I explained that I would open him up from the ribcage to his umbilicus, then I would find a nice, healthy loop of small bowel that could easily be brought up to his stomach. I would align them, open them and suture them together, so that there would be an open avenue for the stomach to drain. It meant that he would be able to eat and drink again, and he could get out of hospital to be at home with his wife and family. Meanwhile, the oncologist had decided that, given the rapidity of progression, Mr O was no longer a candidate for chemotherapy, so this was truly going to be a palliative operation.

I also explained that, as with any operation where we are joining loops of bowel, if the anastomosis did not heal he would leak gastric and small-bowel content into his abdominal cavity, which would make him really sick. At this point, given his cancer prognosis, he would almost certainly not be appropriate for ICU, and he would die.

It was strange to see his eyes twinkle at this thought. As far as he understood, option two was the winner. If the operation was successful, he could eat and drink again; if it was not, this would all be over quickly and without starvation. Both he and his wife decided uniformly that surgery was the best option, and within two hours he was in theatre. Surgery went well, and he returned to the ward with a stomach that could now drain. He recovered slowly, and within days was on his way home, able to eat and drink again freely.

He died eight weeks later. The cancer had continued to progress, obstructing the drainage of bile, and he had become profoundly jaundiced, which in turn had caused his kidneys to fail.

It's funny how everything is relative. Eight weeks at home with family, with the ability to enjoy time – and food – is sometimes a win.

* * *

My mother had been living with me for about seven months by this time, and she was well into her chemotherapy. It was going well and, after the initial shock and upheaval of moving, we had hit a pleasant equilibrium.

My son, in particular, was happy to have his grandmother close to him again. They had a very classic grandmother–grandson relationship, and I was happy for it. As I've mentioned, my mother loved to cook, and my memories of coming home to the smell of biscuits when I was just five were recreated when she baked cinnamon rolls for our morning coffee.

But my mother and I were both shut off to one another. She was instructing from afar my sister, who was running the business at home in order to keep up with bank repayments, but my mother knew she could not share this with me. And

I could not share my work with her. Honestly, I am not sure if anyone can easily share their work with someone non-medical. Maybe they can, but I read somewhere that parents of doctors often do not know what their medical children live through. I also struggled with being both a daughter and a doctor; I just wanted to be a daughter. I did not want to be asked about constipation medications and gripey abdominal pain at home. It had been 15 years since we had last lived together and I think my mother realised that I had flourished in a radically different fashion from my siblings.

One day, I received a voice message on my phone at 5 a.m., and when I replayed it I heard an unfamiliar voice. 'Your sister is here at a hospital in Indonesia. She fell from a waterfall and broke her back. Can you please call us back?' No phone number left to call. This sister, another of the five girls, had been living and working in Sydney.

I tried my sister's phone over and over again. No answer. I started to call hospitals where I thought she might be, but they did not speak English. I knew she would have had travel insurance, so I started to call various travel-insurance companies. I called and called for five hours, until I finally tracked her and her best friend down. My sister had indeed broken her back, but fortunately it was stable and she did not require surgery, although she was in a lot of pain. Unfortunately, the hospital had little staff, and the insurance company would not transfer her without clearance.

So I retrieved her hospital records and X-rays, then sent them to a friend who was a spine surgeon and who, in exchange for a bottle of whisky, wrote a letter to clear her. Finally, the insurance company was willing to transfer her. She would fly to Perth, Australia, where my younger sister (the one who had been back in Samoa working in lieu of my mother) would fly to meet her and look after her while she recuperated from her injury.

My mother cried that entire morning. Probably for fear. Probably for helplessness. When the drama was finally over that afternoon, she came to me with her eyes red. 'Thank you for what you did,' she said.

'Don't worry, Mum,' I replied dismissively, at which she cried some more.

Sometimes, I would look at other families in amazement and wonder what it was like to live in such a seemingly happy and healthy family. What had they done in their lives, I wondered, to deserve such happiness? Of course, the beauty of my job was that it would swiftly put things into perspective. Next thing, I would see a 60-year-old woman who – as well as having a 36-year-old child with severe autism who she could not imagine leaving behind in this world, alone – had a husband dying of cancer for whom she was also the primary caregiver. Then I would realise that maybe my family was not so bad, and I should be grateful.

7.

High-five, nurse!

One morning when I walked into a patient's room, he was educating himself, reading something of a philosophical nature. It was day four of a seven-day stretch of emergency call for me. I had a team in tow: senior registrars about to graduate to consultancy, a few junior registrars aiming to apply for specialty programmes, a couple of house surgeons fresh out of medical school and a medical student. Just like the patient in front of me and the trainee surgeons and medical students around me, I love to learn, and I thrive on philosophical books of this genre. 'Self-help', a friend once described them to me, surprised to find I had quite a selection in my own library. 'Self-enlightenment' is a label I much prefer. I recognised the author of my patient's book, and on the cover, somewhere beneath the title in small print, it read, *Should you trust a doctor who does not look like a doctor?*

I had been the consultant on call the previous night, and the man had been admitted under my care because of abdominal pain. I was amused at his choice of reading material, and his bravery for leaving it there for me to see. I am used to patients telling me I don't look like a surgeon, and I was ready to jump on him. 'So, what does the book say?' I asked, ready for a battle of words.

He looked at me matter-of-factly and directly in the eyes. 'It says that, if you have to choose between a doctor who looks like a doctor and one who does not, choose the one who does not. The one who does not look like a doctor will have had to prove every step of the way that they are just as smart and capable, and will therefore work harder.'

I was very satisfied with this answer, and my smug smile said it all. Our team, diverse in ethnicity and gender, nodded in agreement. Fair play to you, sir.

You might be wondering why this is important. Let me tell you. For a female surgeon to be constantly told that she does not look like a surgeon, or that she is too young to be a surgeon, is significant. Men and women both can be completely befuddled by the idea that women can be surgeons too. My uncle, who lived in the United States and had a niece working as a fully trained surgeon (me), once commented to me that he had been surprised when his own heart surgeon turned out to be a woman. 'So, women *can* be surgeons,' he said – or rather questioned, as if he still required proof. Maybe I have a chip on my shoulder because my father believed that being a good wife was a sufficiently important goal for a woman.

Other common commentary a female surgeon might receive includes, but is not limited to, 'You're the surgeon? But are you a doctor?' and 'Oh, you're a general surgeon? But not a specialist?' Always said as if there must be a missing piece of the puzzle (or, perhaps, anatomy). On one occasion, a patient was confused enough at the end of our bedside visit led by our female professor of surgery to ask when the 'real' professor of surgery was going to visit.

You see, there are many elements that shape the distorted reality of a general surgeon. But, for a woman in training in particular, there are also the many reminders that we are not traditionally seen in the role of surgeon. We continue to be a minority in surgical training. We are frequently reminded by colleagues and patients that we do not, in fact, 'look' like doctors, and even less so like surgeons. My tolerance for this has waned over time. While it may have been laughable when I was a junior doctor, I am in no doubt now that it leads to false assumptions about ability and outcomes.

There are a handful of studies in medical literature that compare patient outcomes, and whether there are differences in death or complication rates, in surgery performed by female surgeons versus male surgeons. One such study, conducted by Wallis et al and published in *The BMJ* in 2017, reported a very small but statistically significant decrease in 30-day mortality for female surgeons compared to male surgeons within a wide spectrum of surgical specialties, including general surgery, neurosurgery and gynaecology.

In other words, if a patient required surgery within any of the aforementioned specialties and their surgeon was a woman, then the study showed they were less likely to die within 30 days of surgery than if their surgeon was a male. For other issues such as a patient's likelihood of developing complications, or the likelihood of being readmitted after surgery, there was no difference between male or female surgeons.

A second, similar study, conducted by Sharoky et al and published in *Annals of Surgery* in 2018, looked at general surgeons performing procedures such as colon or small-bowel resections and cholecystectomies (gallbladder removal). This study found that, after matching female and male surgeons with similar characteristics who treated similar patients at the same hospital, there was no difference in death rates in hospital or complications after surgery, nor in how prolonged the hospital stay was.

In 2017, a large study published by a research group (Y. Tsugawa et al) from Harvard Medical School and the Harvard T.H. Chan School of Public Health reported that, when researchers looked at over 1.5 million hospital admissions for patients 65 years or older, the female internists had statistically significant lower mortality rates than their male counterparts in the same hospital (11.07 per cent versus 11.49 per cent). The difference was small, but when we talk about statistical significance we mean that the result is true and almost certainly not owing to chance.

To elucidate further these differences in outcome depending on whether a surgeon is male or female, a research group from the University of Toronto in Canada conducted by Wallis et al and published in *JAMA Surgery* in 2022 retrieved population data to determine whether surgical outcomes – in particular, poor outcomes, including death, readmission or other complications – were influenced by sex concordance or discordance between surgeon and patient. Put simply, the researchers wanted to examine whether a female patient might have the same outcome whether she was treated by a male surgeon or a female surgeon, and the same examination was also carried out for male patients. They included 21 surgeries from cardiac, vascular, general surgery, urology and orthopaedics. In general surgery, this included appendicectomy, cholecystectomy, gastric bypass, liver resection and colonic resection. The authors found that surgeon–patient gender discordance for female patients with male surgeons resulted in a higher risk of mortality and poor outcomes compared to female patients with female surgeons. This poor outcome for discordance in relation to female patients did not extend to male patients treated by female surgeons; the outcomes in this relationship were comparable or better than a male patient with a male surgeon.

Even the way surgeons are treated by their colleagues differs by gender. A 2017 postdoctoral research paper by Harvard scholar Heather Sarsons examined surgeon gender and how it influenced the way referring physicians interpreted information about a surgeon's ability. It found that, after a patient's death, the perception of skill and ability as evidenced by referrals from colleagues was different depending on whether a surgeon was male or female. If a male surgeon experienced a patient death, he still received more referrals in the time periods following the death relative to the period before. In contrast, a female surgeon received *fewer* referrals after the death than before. The magnitude of difference was such that a male surgeon experienced *three* patient deaths before he had the same reduction in referrals as a female surgeon after *one* death. This difference persisted for a year and a half. Additionally, following the death, patient complexity did not change significantly for male surgeons, but female surgeons received referrals of patients and procedures that were significantly less complex and risky than before.

By comparison, if we look at referral patterns after a good event – meaning a good patient outcome after what is perceived to be incredibly risky surgery – both male and female surgeons received an increase in the number of referrals compared to the period before, but male surgeons received almost twice as many referrals as female surgeons.

* * *

I played a lot of sport as a young woman. One day when I was about 15, I was walking out of the house in my shorts and sports bra when my grandmother stopped me in our living room. 'You should dress so as not to draw a man's eye,' she said.

I was speechless. Momentarily. 'Why is it my responsibility to dress so as not to draw a man's eye? Why is it not the man's responsibility to not look where he should not?'

'A woman has to be modest,' my grandmother replied.

I loved my grandmother. She was loving, and she was a woman of the church. My mother was not so explicit in her expression of a woman's role in society except that she worked hard to make ends meet and did it all with a smile. She could make something out of nothing.

In Samoa, women are chiefs. They dance with fire and knives. They work. They look after the family and rear children, and they always hold their heads high. This is where I learnt a woman's limitless role in society, even if it was not explicitly said. Women are powerful.

* * *

At the time I started writing this book, the surgical society was exploding with the exposure of sexual harassment and bullying. Apparently, no one ever knew or thought that this existed. So, does it?

Several personal experiences come to mind. One of them, the senior consultant who sent me a naked picture of himself while I was in training. The second happened while I was attending a meeting to apply for a specialty programme prior to general surgery. When you apply for a specialty programme, you must spend some time developing yourself into a desirable candidate. This is done through research, introducing yourself to the right people, working hard and attending meetings designed for young trainees and wannabes. This was a weekend meeting, with education during the day and a dinner at night. It was during dinner that one of the consultants put his hand on my leg. Startled, I moved away. 'That's not your leg,' I told him.

Afterwards, I mentioned it to my mentor at the time. 'I wouldn't tell anyone if I were you,' my mentor replied. 'You won't get a job anywhere if you do.' I was stunned at the response, but I knew it to be true. And, besides, what is a hand on the leg? Nothing, I told myself.

Then another colleague I told said, 'You should get it over with, sleep with him, and get onto the programme.'

I was startled by how confronting these conversations were. I decided this programme was not for me, that these particular people would end up being colleagues and this was absolutely not desirable, and I switched codes.

The third and more prolonged experience didn't happen until some years later. I was attending an annual conference, and it had been a long day of lectures and learning. As was usual, a dinner at the end of the day marked a successful event, and allowed for everyone to debrief, network and make new friends. As we exited the restaurant, my boss and supervisor grabbed my shirt roughly. 'I want to fuck you,' he slurred into my ear. I yanked myself free, clung tightly to my friends and left for the safety of my hotel room.

Monday morning came, and so did my boss's clinic, which I was always required to help in. Clinics are often overbooked, and we need all hands on deck to help and keep patients moving. I had never had a problem with him before, but on this particular Monday, three days after he had accosted me, he screamed about how I was incompetent and useless in front of both patients and staff. Ultimately, I tolerated months of this type of aggressive behaviour, including being accused of playing games in front of theatre staff. In response, I chose to focus solely on completing the year, and declined to report him when colleagues suggested I do so. The heat on harassment was on in our industry at that moment, and one colleague was of the opinion that he should be slammed. 'Say the word, and I will get media involved.' Another, a senior colleague, asked if I wanted him to say something.

Of course, my then-supervisor held important positions, which was always going to make it difficult for me, but moreover – and quite bizarrely – I did not want someone slammed, even if he was completely in the wrong. Nor did I want others getting involved and causing trouble for themselves. So, I finished the year, and made sure that, if anything, my position was not reappointed to another person the following year. Then I left.

I have had many a conversation with friends and colleagues since about how I handled this. Some believe I should have complained and done more. The surprising discourse that comes to the surface is the 'correctness' for a consultant to express a romantic or sexual interest in someone who is under his or her supervision. For some, this is acceptable, because one can freely say no. But I can confidently say that the ability to say no from a more junior position, where you rely on your supervisor for education and support, is not a free one. You have to consider how to say no without offending your senior, without jeopardising your chances for a safe and satisfactory working relationship, and without bruising an ego that doesn't tolerate a no. The recipe is not good.

If I had to go back, I am not sure that I would have done anything differently. I was already fighting on several different fronts, and I just wanted to get through my training.

* * *

While on a ward round after a busy 24 hours of acute surgical call, the next patient on our list was a young woman with lower abdominal pain. She was in her twenties and, as is standard, I started with her history – why she had come into hospital, how long she had been in pain, and what made it worse. Also present in the cubicle were the on-call consultant, a fellow registrar and a house surgeon, all of whom happened to be men.

I lifted the patient's gown to examine her, and found she was tender across her entire lower abdomen. 'Your pain is not classic for appendicitis, and your blood tests are normal,' I explained to her. 'I think we should get an ultrasound of your abdomen to look at your ovaries, and then we can see the appendix at the same time.'

Afterwards, the team convened in the central doctors' area, and the consultant spoke up. 'She most likely has chlamydia,' he said, in no uncertain terms. (Chlamydia, for those unfamiliar, is a sexually transmitted infection.) I stared at him in shock, speechless. So he added, 'She has black undies and a belly ring. It's chlamydia.'

I immediately thought of the black lacy underwear that I, too, had donned that morning and of my belly ring, not to mention my back tattoo, and I was quick to tell him that my own vaginal swabs had come back clear of chlamydia just last week. I was incensed at his derogatory comments – that they were made in front of me, yes, but even more so in front of young male staff who might find such discriminatory assessments acceptable.

Oblivious of the benefit to women, this same consultant decided some time after this event that he would no longer see female patients with haemorrhoids, because women were too difficult.

And, by the way, the young woman did not have chlamydia.

* * *

As I walked through a four-bed cubicle during one of my morning rounds, I was perturbed to find a man in his bed with the curtain open. These four-bed cubicles leave no dignity for those who dare to cross their threshold – patients and surgeons alike. There is no privacy and all laundry is aired.

This man had been given an inch and was taking a mile. He was obese, and probably in his fifties, but it was difficult to see why he had been admitted. Sometimes, we can tell by intelligent examination of the surroundings – for example, if he'd had one healthy-looking leg and the other was absent from the knee down, a stump swathed with bandages, I would have ascertained that he was a diabetic who had come in with a dead leg requiring amputation. Or, if he was thin or malnourished with a big bag of nutrition being infused through his veins, and perhaps a tube out of his nose, then he might have had Crohn's disease (a chronic disease of the gastrointestinal tract). This man had both his legs, and definitely did not have a problem with malnutrition.

He was lying on his side with his knees splayed apart. 'Doctor!' he shouted as I walked past. Naively, I turned my head to look, and it was then that he lifted his gown, exposed his genitalia and asked me to wash his balls.

This is not uncommon. I have had many female colleagues share similar stories. Full credit to the nursing staff, who probably have to deal with this sort of behaviour endlessly. However, I have always wondered if a female patient would expose herself in the same way and ask a male surgeon to douche her vagina. I would be more than happy to be corrected, but I can only assume not.

* * *

Back when I was still undecided about my choice of surgical specialty, I was attached as a junior resident to a male consultant who seemed interested in what I might choose to practise long-term. The fact that a senior consultant was interested in my future plans was very flattering. We were standing over the scrub basin, washing our hands in tandem between cases. Often these moments can be awkward, especially if you have nothing to share. The days can be long.

'What will you do?' he asked, as he used his elbow to dispense more of the brown cleansing solution.

'Either urology or general surgery. I'm not quite sure yet,' I told him confidently. I was young and bright-eyed, a firm believer that the world really was my oyster.

There was a short silence, and then he filled it. 'If you want my opinion, women should just do what men have been doing for years, and choose between a family or a career. The problem with women these days is that they want it all.'

I was floored. I knew he had a faithful wife, who managed his private practice, and four beautiful daughters. How could he say that? How could he say that *he* had chosen one or the other, when it was clearly a choice he had never had to make?

He had both his family and a career. I meekly pointed out that perhaps I, too, needed his wife. He raised his eyebrows, and we continued our day in theatre.

The case was a challenging one. It was a breast-surgery attachment, and we were operating on breast cancers that day. Breasts can be very vascular, meaning that they can bleed a lot. Fortunately, it is usually easy to control. This woman had particularly pendulous breasts and she was bleeding briskly, which was to be expected. 'Women have more blood supply to their breasts than to their brains,' the consultant said as he turned to me.

Misogynist was the first word that came to my mind. Arsehole was the next.

* * *

Four highly skilled female surgical registrars were on duty over a weekend, from Friday to Monday. As per expectations, they visited every single patient on every single one of those days. They assessed patients, operated, reviewed results, re-reviewed patients and discharged, as one normally does while on call. The weekend was unremarkable. Busy, but they were efficient and it passed smoothly.

Less than two weeks later, the head of department approached the senior female registrar to discuss an official complaint that had been lodged by a female patient. Said patient had been admitted over the weekend, and during that weekend claimed to have only been reviewed by nursing staff. She was, she reported, shocked and dismayed to have been discharged from hospital on Monday morning by a nurse. And she was even more shocked that, at no point during her admission, was she reviewed by a doctor. A strange complaint indeed. Even stranger was the fact that she did not raise her concern during her admission or before she was sent out the door with her suitcase.

The senior registrar, a good friend, was irate. She recalled the patient, and recalled very clearly assessing her on the ward round. To be doubly sure, my friend checked the medical records. The clinical notes documented that this patient had been seen every single day of her admission by all four female surgical registrars, and the most senior registrar had discharged her on the Monday.

The head of department, a lovely Englishman, well dressed in his suit and red tie chided the female registrars condescendingly. 'You need to identify yourselves more clearly as doctors,' he said. I actually witnessed this little dance of fire in the hospital corridor, and I still laugh thinking about it. As my jaw dropped at his patronising response, and before the next words out of my mouth could be 'What the fuck?', my friend jumped in. 'Every time I see a patient, I identify myself as a surgical doctor,' she responded heatedly, but appropriately. 'I have doctor on my badge. I have doctor on my scrubs. I have doctor on my scrub hat. I have doctor on my ID card. What I really need is to walk in with a big dick in my hand.' She was, unfortunately, absolutely right! The head of department laughed nervously. It must be a tough job dealing with hysterical women. Pleonasm for him, I suspect.

One day while reviewing a scan between theatre cases, I rushed to the radiology department in my surgical scrubs to see one of the specialty radiologists. She was a woman, but more importantly an amazing radiologist. There we were having a professional conversation behind closed doors about an MRI in order to plan my breast-cancer operating list the following week when we were interrupted by a male colleague throwing open the door. He had his flock in tow – an array of junior doctors and medical students – and they were totally in awe of his bravado. 'Are you done gossiping?' he asked loudly. 'I need to review a scan.' Of course, two women behind closed doors could not possibly be talking about work.

* * *

It comes as no surprise that, in 1991, a survey of physicians published in the *Journal of Behavioral Medicine* found that women were more likely to leave because of workplace issues – things like control over one's medical or surgical practice, the opportunity for advancement (or lack thereof) and harassment. There is often a perception that women are more likely to leave because of the stress and conflict between personal and professional lives, but in fact the survey found that these levels of conflict were somewhat similar across both genders.

Of course, medicine has come a long way since the '90s, but there are many barriers to women in surgery, and there is much work being done to better understand just what they are (De Costa 2018; Bellini 2019; Liang 2019). In 1970, only 8 per cent of physicians were female, and they constituted 13 per cent of the undergraduate medical school. The feminisation of medicine, as Jodi Paik referred to it in her 2000 article by the same name, has seen this proportion increase to an equal 50:50 split for men and women entering medical training. A huge change. Yet, even when women are accepted onto surgical programmes, they have higher rates of attrition, citing reasons such as lack of flexibility and inadequate role models (Bellini 2019; Mitchell 2014). Of course, there are many barriers that are not easily measurable, but the recruitment of women into surgery and into consultant positions is an important goal. In surgery, we see approximately 20 to 30 per cent of females occupying consultant surgeon positions, with minor differences by country and much larger differences by specialty. Regardless, gender seems to be deeply entrenched in the ideal surgeon phenotype.

Midway through her pregnancy, a healthy colleague was still working full-time as a surgeon when she was asked to refer a case for a second opinion. This is not unusual. Indeed, it is encouraged – if you want a second opinion, you are entitled to it. What came as a surprise was the reason the second opinion was sought: her pregnancy, and therefore her ability to think clearly and operate safely, was apparently a cause for concern. She was stunned, but made the referral to a surgeon who did not have a uterus, nonetheless.

Any objective evidence for so-called 'baby brain' is mixed, and of course the quality of the evidence is poor. Some studies say there is significant cognitive decline, while others say there is not. In 2018, a study was published which combined the results of available literature examining differences in cognitive function for pregnant and non-pregnant women. The study reported that pregnant women fared worse than their non-pregnant counterparts across all spectrums – general cognition, memory, executive functioning and attention. The author went on to say that these results needed to be interpreted with caution because the studies themselves were limited, the combined differences were small to moderate, and even then the scores for pregnant women were still within the range of normal. More importantly, they reinforced that these differences are likely to be most noticeable to the woman herself, and there is no evidence that it affects her professional abilities.

Disappointingly, even colleagues in training are moulded by the same societal constructs that have long governed gender. A female junior doctor who openly expressed her desire to specialise in surgery in the shared offices one day was promptly asked by a male colleague if she had considered her unborn children. 'It is a selfish decision for your future family,' he volunteered unwelcomely. Was a man ever told the same thing?

One weekend while I was the consultant on call, we had five on the rounding team, and the senior registrar happened to have a lovely, dense beard, fashionable spectacles and kind eyes. I must say, he looked wise. We stood around the bed of our first patient, an elderly woman with abdominal pain. Her investigations were normal, and I was going to let her go home. Standing to her right, which is where the lead of the round should stand, I explained what we had found, examined her, then told her she could call her husband to collect her. It was obvious she was more reassured by the senior registrar than by me, because she kept directing questions his way and looking at him for confirmation of what I was saying. The source of her confusion became clear as we exited the cubicle. 'Excuse me, miss,' she said to me. 'Can you please butter my toast?' She asked so kindly that I did as she asked – I even put jam on it.

Not so long ago, I was reminded of this when a female registrar came to speak with me in the theatre tearoom. At the end of a long round, we often take time over coffee to summarise our patients – what they need to have done, who will do it, and the priority of those things. She had just come from the ward, where she had been finishing a patient review, and before she could exit the cubicle another irate patient had walked up to her and demanded a cup of tea. 'How do you take your tea, ma'am?' the registrar asked politely.

'What kind of kitchen do you run in this place? I've already told your staff: milk, no sugar.'

Some days the stereotype is funny, but some days it is not.

* * *

When my son was six years old, attentive to fairy tales and modern literature like many young children, he drew a picture of me as a nurse. I was standing next to a doctor, who was a man. Normal. 'You know, it is your mother who is the doctor,' I told him.

'Women can be doctors?' he exclaimed in surprise.

'Yes, they can,' I replied. 'Anyone can be anything they want.'

And, the next time I picked him up from basketball practice, I heard him saying to his friends, 'My mum is a doctor. Did you know women can be doctors, too?'

* * *

A few weeks after the complaint directed at my friend, I was the surgeon on acute call for the week when a young female was admitted with acute cholecystitis. Her gallbladder had stones and was inflamed. She would be best treated with an emergency keyhole operation to remove the gallbladder, because she was almost certainly going to have another attack in the near future, and it would have an effect on her work, family and general quality of life.

Our morning ward rounds could be impressive because of the number of people in the group – everybody is contributing or learning or both. This morning ward round was no different. I led the team in to see this young woman, and went to stand directly on her right, introducing myself as the surgeon on call before introducing the rest of the team, who stood at the foot of her bed writing notes, checking her nursing documentation from the night, updating any prescriptions on her drug chart, checking her blood tests from the day before, and putting new forms out for blood tests to check trends. There was only one man in the team – the fellow, which is to say he had completed his surgical training and was a consultant, but required further specialty training before practising independently.

I explained to the patient that she needed surgery, why she needed surgery, what would happen if she did not have surgery, and the risks and benefits of the procedure. We scheduled her for surgery on our emergency list later that afternoon, and the next time I saw her she was asleep on the operating table. Surgery was uncomplicated, and I reviewed her again in recovery. She had some pain, and I reassured her that the operation had gone well and that we would make her comfortable. Her husband was by her side, and I reassured them both. In fact, I was pretty proud of just how much reassuring I was doing. I was almost patting myself on the back.

The following morning, I saw her again, with the team, to explain what we had found. I told her I was very happy with how the procedure had gone, and that I was confident she would do well and could go home safely. She was elated. We love to make our patients happy.

'High-five, nurse!' she said as she raised her hand.

There was dead silence from the team – the five female doctors dejectedly exchanged glances, while the only man had a look of embarrassment on his bearded face and refused to meet our eyes.

8.

All in a day's work

Sometimes, you cannot predict a patient's response. You might work tirelessly for a patient who flies through treatment without batting an eyelid and get a complaint at the end, or you might have a major complication and be bowled over with gratitude, or you might perform the simplest of procedures and change someone's life.

When one man came in with an acute bowel obstruction, I had to operate on him urgently, but unfortunately he had a major complication and required secondary surgery, before ending up in intensive care. Despite this, his family gifted us generously, and were so appreciative of the care we gave him. Their gratitude made me feel even worse than I already did because of his complicated recovery.

One of my most grateful patients was a woman in her forties who, since having her first child 20 years previously, had struggled with haemorrhoids that dropped out of her anal canal. Haemorrhoids are vascular cushions that are found at the top of the anal canal. They are thought to confer a degree of faecal continence, and can be symptomatic for a number of reasons. For some people, they can be horribly problematic; for a general surgeon, they are one of our commonest clinic complaints. If they ulcerate, they can cause rectal bleeding, which usually shows as bright red blood found on toilet paper when wiping after a bowel motion. At their worst, they can bleed constantly and lead to anaemia, or they can become so big that they prolapse out of the anal canal and continue to become engorged, causing immense pain. The latter is not a pretty sight. This woman's haemorrhoids were sometimes small, sometimes fuller. It all depended on what her diet and stress levels had been like, and whether she was engaging in her normal daily routines. With each of her three pregnancies, her haemorrhoids had become worse, but she rallied through each of them.

When she finally found the time to get help, she asked her GP to refer her to us for an intervention. She needed surgery both because of the size of the haemorrhoids and the amount of tissue involved. This is one of my least favourite operations, primarily because it can be an uphill battle to get your patient through the recovery. As you can imagine, any trauma in and around the anal canal is incredibly painful. It is also incredibly difficult to clean and nurse. Even though I always warned patients of the pain after surgery, I found that I could never warn them enough about how difficult recovery would be. Most, if not all, were surprised at how sore they were, and how long they remained that way. However, this lady rallied through the recovery – the three children and size of the haemorrhoids gave us a clue – and sent us boxes of exquisite chocolates with cards telling us how we had made wiping her arse the most pleasurable it had been in 20 years.

Sometimes we do not know what bad is until we are good again.

* * *

If the abdomen is bound above by the ribcage, and below by oblique lines running from the hip bones to the pubic bone, then it is further divided into ninths by straight lines running from the mid-point of each clavicle above and bisected by two transverse lines. The first of these lines is halfway between the jugular notch – the palpable dip at the top of the breastbone and the pubic symphysis – and the second line runs horizontally between each of the anterior prominences of the hips.

Dividing the abdomen into nine segments in this way allows us to think systematically about the organs that might be causing a symptomatic presentation. If pain is around the umbilicus (belly button), it might be the small bowel causing the trouble. If it is in the right uppermost segment, it might be the liver. Mrs O, a fit and well woman in her fifties, presented with pain in her right iliac fossa, the lowermost right segment that houses the appendix – and also, for women, the ovaries and fallopian tube.

Mrs O had been sent to us to exclude an appendicitis. We know that people's bodies can do funny things, and not all pathologies go by the book, but she had a somewhat atypical presentation for appendicitis based on the duration of her symptoms and her ability to move around comfortably. Her CT scan demonstrated an acute appendicitis, but with a large phlegmon (inflammation of soft tissue) around it.

This meant that surgery was going to be difficult, because an inflammatory mass often has other loops of bowel stuck to it, increasing the risk of damage to adjacent structures when trying to remove the appendix. In addition, appendicectomy is standardly performed as a laparoscopic procedure, but the chance that she would require an open operation instead was significantly higher than if this had been an early appendicitis without a big inflammatory mass. It also increased the chance that we would have to take more bowel than was necessary. Therefore, we opted to nurse her with antibiotics to settle the inflammation first, and planned to remove the appendix some weeks later. If we could be sure the inflammatory mass was settled, the operation to remove her appendix would have the best chance of being completed laparoscopically, with minimal risk of damage to adjacent structures.

In the interim, Mrs O kept us regularly informed, detailing how much she was struggling with her recovery, despite paying excessive attention to her diet and sensation of wellness. She was miserable on antibiotics and, because she was not 100 per cent, she could not go about her normal daily activities. When she came to see us after eight weeks of careful non-operative management, she was in tears.

'But what's wrong?' I asked. 'You look in great shape.' I meant it.

'It's terrible, Dr Meredith,' she said with gravity. 'We have too many houses, and I am finding it quite stressful thinking about what to do with them all.'

First World problems, then.

* * *

Pancreatitis is a very common diagnosis on surgical wards. A patient presents with vomiting and pain in the upper abdomen that radiates through to their back. The pancreas sits behind the stomach, and the two most common reasons for inflammation in this gland are alcohol and gallstones – excluding countries where scorpion stings are common, in which case these might be in the top two. As surgeons, we simply manage a pancreatitic patient with supportive care – intravenous fluids and pain relief – and wait for them to settle. Pancreatitis can be mild and require only pain relief, or it can be severe enough to require intensive care support or even cause death.

Mrs G was a wealthy woman in her sixties who was accompanied by her husband. They had played a wonderful round of golf that sunny day, but she had developed increasing abdominal pain with each successive hole, and by the end of it she was in agony. They came to hospital dressed in their classy tweed golf attire, and when we walked into her cubicle she lay perfectly in her bed while he read his luxury watch magazine.

As usual, I started with an open-ended question so she could tell me from the beginning about her complaint and the evolution of it. I had already seen her blood tests and her X-rays and scans. Her blood tests showed she had a pancreatitis, and this was confirmed by her history and examination. She did not have gallstones, but they had given a dinner party the night before, and had consumed perhaps a little more alcohol than they would normally.

'What did you drink?' I asked.

'Brandy. We always drink brandy,' she replied.

I explained that it looked as if the pancreatitis episode might have been caused by alcohol, given that we had excluded all other causes and that the episode followed their dinner party. This upset both of them greatly.

'Can she ever drink alcohol again?' her husband asked with a worried look on his face.

'Unfortunately, there is no threshold over which we can accurately predict when she might develop pancreatitis,' I replied, then reiterated that this was a mild episode, but that people can be severely ill or die with it. Sometimes our best recommendation in such a scenario is abstinence, I explained, but obviously a patient has to make their own decisions.

She listened to all this, and said she would try to negotiate a safe amount of alcohol that she could drink on a daily basis.

'I'm sorry I can't be more helpful with regard to the amount of alcohol you can drink safely,' I said, 'but it seems this episode will settle quickly, and you should be able to go home in the next twenty-four to forty-eight hours.'

We said goodnight, and I left the room.

A moment later, her husband ran out after us, having just remembered an important detail. We stopped in the hallway to hear what he wanted to add. 'We usually drink French brandy. Very expensive French brandy,' he said. 'But we ran out and had to drink a much cheaper brand. Could that be why she has the pancreatitis?'

'I don't think so, sir,' I heard my registrar reply.

* * *

A 35-year-old woman came to see me in clinic with an anal problem. The referral letter said that she had a large fleshy growth at the anal verge, and it was impairing her ability to work. I could understand that a large fleshy growth at the anus would impair one's ability to work. It sounded awfully uncomfortable. We had a brief conversation about how long it had been there, if it was causing her pain and if it was bleeding. Then I asked to examine her, and instructed her how to position herself on the examination table: pants down to her knees, buttocks placed exactly at the edge of the table so they are just hanging off it, right shoulder forward, knees to her chest and feet forward. It is always a delight when someone is limber enough to position themselves like this independently. For a man in his eighties with a stiff back, it is never easy or quick.

I spread her buttocks apart in search of the large fleshy growth, but was disappointed to find a tiny little tag at what I would call the 12 o'clock position. She had a bit of extra flesh at the top of the anal verge, just behind the perineum. I completed a thorough check to make sure I was not missing anything. Gloves, lubricant jelly over the index finger, gentle internal examination of the anal canal, digital rectal examination, then a tube to examine the rectum and another tube to look inside the anal canal and check for haemorrhoids. The examination revealed no other findings. Just this small, pathetic bit of extra tissue at 12 o'clock.

'Is this what you are worried about?' I asked her. 'I would leave that well alone.' I then went on to explain that the procedure to remove the tag was not worth the trouble because it was so small and it was benign. It was barely worth mentioning.

'But I can't work,' she said.

'What work do you do?' I asked.

'I am a high-end escort and I've been losing work because of this.'

I pushed down my absolute astonishment and, although I definitely did not see how she could be losing work because of this tiny tag, I filled out the booking for an excision under anaesthetic.

* * *

It was back when I was a registrar in urology that I had first become aware of nether-region preoccupations. In particular, I discovered that some men seem to like placing foreign bodies in their urethra – the tube that runs from the tip of the penis to the bladder. Men ejaculate and urinate through this hole. Why would someone want to push solid objects up there? One man let barely a day go by after being sent home before he put his toothbrush back into his penis – and not handle first. This guy's penis had been forced to swallow a toothbrush whole, brush first. Why? But, even more importantly, why not the handle first? Still, maybe he was marginally saner than the razor-blade guy. Yes, razor blades into the penis. Do not ask me how, or why.

In general surgery, it is more common to encounter foreign bodies in the rectum. This was a highlight for all young surgical registrars, largely because of the storytelling. Most of the time, the foreign body is retrievable simply by putting the victim to sleep – thanks to the anaesthetist – so that the voluntary sphincter mechanism of the anus no longer puts up a fight. I can honestly say I never had a female patient present with a rectal foreign body, whereas the male is a true victim because he has usually just been walking through the house minding his own business. It is always so unfortunate that he was going down the stairs naked and unaware of the

158

Barbie doll lurking at the bottom until he slipped and fell on top of her. Or that the broom was standing upright when he slipped from the porch. Or that there were knitting needles standing on the bathroom floor when he hopped out of the shower. I learnt that some homes are incredibly dangerous, especially for men walking around naked in the presence of fruits and vegetables, light bulbs and jars. Stairs are the worst. You never know what is lying, or standing, at the bottom of them.

Mr GP (for Great Party) had come from one. He was in his twenties and presented as a little confused. He had been at said great party the night before, and now more than 12 hours later entered the acute assessment unit dressed casually in jeans and a T-shirt.

'What brings you to hospital?' the registrar asked. This was the sort of standard, open-ended question we are taught in medical school to ask so as to allow the patient to partake freely in the discourse.

'I think I have vegetables in my rectum,' the man replied.

After a moment of unimpressed silence (the days are difficult enough without people trying to be mysterious), the registrar repeated, 'You think you have vegetables in your rectum?'

'Yes,' the young man said, as if it was of no consequence, and apparently unwilling to divulge more than was asked of him, even though he had presented voluntarily to the hospital.

'What makes you think that you have vegetables in your rectum?' the registrar asked patiently.

'I went to a party last night, and some vegetables went missing.'

More silence.

'What vegetables went missing?' the registrar asked.

'A cucumber and a carrot.'

'And what makes you think they are in your rectum?' (Sometimes, it is like pulling teeth.)

'I don't remember the end of the party. All I know is that vegetables went missing because I counted them before, and I am pretty sure they are in my rectum.'

Yet another innocent victim of a cucumber. It was not even a full moon.

* * *

I could write excessively about rectums and bowel motions because I've seen a lot of both as a general surgeon. We are called for constipation, diarrhoea and overly offensive stools. Sometimes, the smell follows us home. It sticks to our skin, our nostrils and even crosses the flimsy barrier of a latex glove. I was mortified during one busy general surgical clinic when, somewhere in among the new consultations for rectal bleeding, a patient commented that I must have been doing my job for a long time, because I had just inserted first my finger and then a cold tube into his rectum without telling him. I was shocked, and profusely apologetic. Apparently I had just flipped into automatic-pilot mode and done a complete examination of his rectum for bleeding. Had we even had a conversation?

Rostered on a night shift, a friend and I were taking turns seeing patients as they came through the door. Night shifts are horrible, but sharing them with friends can make all the difference, especially if you plan a boozy breakfast for the morning. The next woman who came through triage was complaining of abdominal pain, and it was my friend's turn. The woman had routine bloods and X-rays done, and a rectal examination. There is a saying that if you don't put your finger in it, you will put your foot in it. So, my friend put his gloves on and, with his patient positioned appropriately, inserted a gloved digit into her anal canal. He felt nothing abnormal. No rectal masses. Soft motions in the rectum. Anal canal normal. Sufficient medical documentation for a rectal examination.

Through the window of the cubicle, I saw my friend exit the examination area and proceed to deglove at the basin. Then I saw him jumping about in distress and mouthing numerous expletives. I poked my head through the door to see if all was okay. He dry-wretched as he showed me his bare hand, his entire index finger covered in brown stool. It had even got underneath his fingernail. The glove had a hole in it. Add to the medical notes: *Brown stool. No blood.*

* * *

Sometimes, the monotony of rectal exams and bowel motions is broken up by other important aspects of general surgery, such as other body parts. I was in a routine breast clinic with a new patient who unfortunately did not speak English. These consults are always tough, because communication is completely unsatisfactory for both parties. She was elderly, in her eighties, and accompanied by her daughter, who spoke English only marginally better and unfortunately not well enough to convey the nature of the problem.

I asked the elderly woman to sit on the side of the bed and remove her shirt and bra, but her presenting problem was still not clear. It was a breast clinic, however, and her primary care physician had referred her for a nipple problem, so at least she was in the right place. She was slight, her breasts a little empty, consistent with her frame and having breastfed in the long-distant past. A thorough examination ensued, and I could find no abnormality.

After a futile attempt at a mixture of broken English and unofficial sign language, I was still in the dark. I decided to perform a second examination. I leaned my head a little closer to the woman's chest, in an investigative manner, then lifted her floppy left breast. In doing so, I squeezed the tissue behind her nipple, which was directly in line with my eye. I could not duck fast enough when pus exploded from the tiny openings in the nipple, and before I knew it my face was covered in breast pus.

'Yes! Yes! Yes!' shouted the patient's daughter.

* * *

Let's call him Mr A for good measure. This fit and well man in his forties was having trouble with rectal prolapse, or so he thought. Rectal prolapse is where the rectum literally descends through the anus. No small social problem. However, this man did not fit any of the at-risk features for prolapse. He was young, with no medical problems, and more likely had been having trouble with large haemorrhoids, a far easier problem to fix.

Nonetheless, a practical man and carpenter by profession, Mr A had decided one Saturday morning he needed to fix the problem. He was strong and well built, a typical no-nonsense New Zealand bloke. He knew the local hardware store opened at 6.30 a.m. and stocked anything the do-it-yourself fixer-upper might need because he had cruised those aisles many times before. I suppose any reliable builder considering the problem at hand – an incompetent rectum that drops out into the underwear through the anus – would desire something durable and solid to reinforce the rectal walls ... but, of course, whatever the chosen form of reinforcement, it had to traverse the anus first. Perhaps, then, something in liquid form? Something that becomes solid after accurate placement?

The lightbulb moment that ensued was unfortunate for Mr A. Concrete and the rectum are not compatible. The immensity of their incompatibility became obvious shortly after installation.

Even worse, a good general anaesthetic and a pair of gloves was not enough to retrieve this foreign body. The chemical reaction and the pressure had burned through the wall of his rectum, and he required an emergency operation to resect the unhealthy rectum, en bloc with the concrete, and bring his bowel out to the abdominal wall, where his faeces would deposit themselves into a bag that he would have to empty twice a day.

Suffice to say, he will no longer have trouble with rectal prolapse.

* * *

After having escaped a drug raid, Mr D arrived at the emergency department looking panicked and dishevelled. That morning, the cops and their canines had knocked his door down and disrupted his sweet reveries.

The liquid ecstasy in his cupboard jolted him into action. He placed every drop he had into the nearest jar, pushed it up his anus with brute force and jumped out of the window. Then, worried that he might disrupt his insides, Mr D headed straight for the hospital and asked the kind doctors in the emergency department for assistance. Unfortunately, the surgeons had to be called in for this one. 'What exactly did you put up there? How big? Do you have any medical problems?' Standard questions, but the answers didn't change the outcome. He still required a general anaesthetic. He was a thin guy with greasy hair and an air of nervousness about him, but who could blame him? He was probably ashamed of what we were about to find.

Sleeping peacefully under a general anaesthetic, and far away in a land of dreams without the police breaking down his front door, he was in the standard position for foreign-body retrieval from his rectum: flat on his back with his legs in stirrups. We were surprised when a gloved finger into the rectum demonstrated just how big the jar was. Grabbing it was difficult. It would not budge. The male pelvis can be very narrow, as Mr D's was, and the jar had firmly lodged itself in the warm embrace of his pelvic walls. Fingers and even the smallest hands failed, as did both the forceps and ventouse vacuum normally used to grab a baby's head during a difficult vaginal delivery.

Time passed, and another specialist was called to theatre to assist. The big guns. This surgeon was the rectum specialist. Still no luck. The decision was then made to open Mr D's abdomen, make a hole in his rectum and retrieve the jar that way. This time, success!

Much to our horror, he had used a well-secured 250-millilitre jar. The maths did not quite add up – a few drops of liquid ecstasy in a huge jar stuffed up his anus seemed somewhat Darwinian. And, much to his horror, he woke with a far bigger scar than he'd anticipated and no doubt a very sore anus.

Plans were made to see him again in a few weeks, largely to assess his continence. With all the handling and instrumentation, we were worried. Surely he would have trouble holding onto his faeces with a disrupted sphincter.

Alas, he has not been seen since.

* * *

Mrs C, a frail woman in her seventies, came to the clinic because she was suffering from intractable constipation. She sat down in the chair facing me and put a spoon on my desk. 'What's this for?' I asked.

'I need to use this to evacuate my bowels every day,' she said without hesitation.

I found myself struggling for words. 'How?' I finally managed.

'I use this end of the spoon to scoop out my faeces.' She pointed to the wide, round end that we usually put into the other end of the alimentary tract.

'You should take that and put it back in your bag,' I told her.

'I clean it after every use,' she said, as if there was nothing strange about what she was saying.

'Please, just put it away.' I was envisioning her morning routine, and made a conscious decision not to ask whether

166

she ever put the spoon back in the kitchen drawer with all the other cutleries. And, even though I had not touched it, I found myself reaching for the hand sanitiser.

To be fair, I was still recovering from the previous patient, who had brought in a container of her blood-covered faeces following her morning coffee. There is something very unique about the way many humans need to prove what comes out of their anus, lumps and all. I can honestly say that I have never seen such a consistent obsession with lumps or discharge from any other part of the body. People bring in evidence of their motions without hesitation. They also take photographs of their anuses quite readily. Smartphones have certainly changed society, no matter your age.

* * *

My junior colleague, the house surgeon, wanted to specialise in surgery, so on a busy weekend decided she would help us see acute patients. The next patient we'd been called to assist was a young man admitted to the orthopaedic ward. He had sustained spinal trauma after a dirt-bike accident and, as is often the case after trauma and in someone on bed rest and strong pain relief, his bowels had stopped working.

The house surgeon diligently took his story, asked if there was anything else we needed to know about his bowel history, then examined his abdomen and took X-rays. Her assessment was a pseudo-obstruction, meaning that his body was behaving as if he had an obstructed bowel, but rather than being truly mechanical (for instance, because of a cancer) it was the result of many factors: the trauma, the bed rest and the constipation-inducing narcotics to keep him comfortable. He required a tube in his rectum, and at the same time the house surgeon would look inside his rectum with a rigid scope.

This is a trap for enthusiastic general surgery wannabes. We have all been characters in stories such as this one. The house surgeon, with the help of one of the nurse aides, positioned her patient for his rectal examination. However, the routine rectal intubation position – lying on the left side, knees to the chest and buttocks as close to the edge of the bed as can be – was not possible in a patient with trauma such as this. The house surgeon made do, however. She lubricated the end of the rigid scope and inserted it into his anus. There are two parts to the rigid scope: the blunt tube with which to insufflate, and inside that the tapered tube, which makes entry into the anal canal a little easier for the surgeon and much more pleasant for the patient. Once sufficiently introduced, the internal tapered tube is removed so that you can look through the glass window on the blunt tube. The house surgeon had her head by the glass window of the rectal scope when she removed the inside tube – an amateur mistake. The patient's colon was full of air and, under pressure, it was ready to be decompressed through the path of least resistance. Faeces exploded all over the house surgeon's face, hair and arms, not to mention the curtains and wall behind her. She ran to the sluice and vomited.

There is that saying, 'Some days the pigeon, and some days the statue.' In general surgery, one must always be ready to be the statue.

* * *

Thirty-four-year-old Mr M was a well-built man with a few tattoos for extra measure. Every time he passed a bowel motion, it was coated in bright-red blood, which also made its way onto the toilet paper. He had no weight loss and no family history of bowel cancer, both reassuring pieces of information, and it was likely his problem was benign. Examination confirmed this: he had a couple of simple haemorrhoids. Not terribly exciting.

A couple of rubber bands would fix them easily. Much like docking a sheep's tail, placing a rubber band tightly at the base of the haemorrhoid strangles the blood supply so that it eventually shrivels away. Haemorrhoids are situated at the junction between skin where we are incredibly sensitive to pain and the mucosa, which lines the inside of the gut and our mouths and is generally insensate. It is therefore important when placing the rubber bands to put them where there is no sensation – that is, above the level of the skin.

We got Mr M into position, lying on his side, pants round his knees, bottom hanging over the edge of the bed and proctoscope traversing his anus. It's a position reproduced and perfected over many years, and often requires the help of a wonderful clinic nurse. It is surprisingly complex to achieve.

'I can't feel a thing,' Mr M said when the suction catheter was rested on the base of a haemorrhoid, leading the surgeon to believe that the catheter was above the skin and safely on mucosa. The first band went on, and Mr M winced.

'Did you feel that?' his surgeon enquired.

'Nope,' he replied, probably a little too quickly.

The second band went on. Mr M winced again.

'I'm going to get you some Panadol,' said his surgeon.

Less than ten minutes passed after applying Mr M's bands before screaming was heard from the corridor. 'Help me! Somebody help me!' He was found on all fours on the floor just outside a packed waiting room, still with his pants round his knees, sweating and crying. 'Help me!' he cried one more time before he fell flat on his face. His bare arse was facing the sky and he had stopped breathing.

Stunned at this incredible turn of events, it took a moment for the team to click into action. As for any arrest call, nurses and doctors flocked from every room, and the crash-cart trolley rolled down the hall. CPR ensued and Mr M was taken straight to the operating theatre to have his bands removed. The haemorrhoids could wait for another day.

Maybe Mike Tyson was right. Everyone has a plan until they get punched in the mouth.

9.

Patience and wisdom

I believe the discovery of my pregnancy at 26 weeks happened for a reason. It brought me close to my mother again, and kept me close to the family. However, since surgical training required me to move frequently, my son and I had changed neighbourhoods, cities, schools and countries all before he was 13.

When he was 12, we moved to Sydney so that I could begin training in breast-cancer reconstruction. While still in my first general consultant year and deciding on my subspecialty of choice, I'd had the chance to attend the American College of Surgeons annual congress and it was there I realised that, above all else, I enjoyed accompanying people on their journey to be cancer-free. My mother had finished her chemotherapy by this time, and was travelling between New Zealand and Samoa for check-ups. I felt that I identified with the shared fight for best possible outcomes, and I also felt that I understood the impact that cancer had on families more than many of my colleagues. And so I fell into the world of breast-cancer surgery and reconstruction.

My son never kicked up a fuss. He was incredibly adaptable, but sometimes I think he grew up alone. By the time he was 11, I was leaving him on his own at the house whenever I had to return to theatre or see a patient in the emergency department. Before heading out the door, I would reiterate the rules: 1) do not let anyone in the house, not even friends, because then they will know that you are alone and you are not supposed to be alone (usually followed by 'and you do not want me to go to prison, do you?'), and 2) do not call me unless there is an emergency.

I love my son, and I believe that my key role on this earth is to make sure he is the best that he can possibly be. My siblings joked that he was a trust-fund baby because I would give him everything he wanted. Eager for him to have the life that I had not, I enrolled him in any sport or activity that I could. Thousands of dollars were spent on football, swimming, basketball, tennis, surf lifesaving and guitar lessons.

Even so, in my opinion, I did not do enough for him, and I was always absent. But it was just us two. His father was out of the picture and had very little input into his son's life. So, I was mother *and* father, wrapped up in one angry person. Meanwhile, my son was so gentle that it frightened me. My perception of society was that one had to fight and experience pain to be where they wanted to be, but this was not his perception at all.

One day when he was about 11, I was watching one of his basketball games, and I still don't understand precisely what happened except that I noticed a kid from the opposing team was throwing offenses at my son and being needlessly aggressive. My son came off the court in tears. 'I want to go home,' he said.

'Why?' I asked, probably unfairly.

'I just want to go home.'

'No way. I am not taking you home,' I said. 'I see what is happening. You get back on that court and you give back to that kid.'

'I don't want to. I want to go home.'

'I don't care what you want to do. I am not taking you home until you get back on that court and fight for yourself.'

The coach walked over, a lovely lady who had been part of my afterschool childcare plan. 'Uh, Ineke,' she started uncomfortably, 'you can both go home now.'

I smiled stiffly and waited for half-time. On my way out, I found 'the kid'. 'You should be careful,' I told him. 'One day someone will come back for you, and you will regret being a little shit.' Then I took my son home.

He was a gifted swimmer, and trained with a squad run by a South African lady who had coached her surf-lifesaving team to international success. I hated to watch these training sessions because they looked so painful: the 11-year-old kids were made to swim lap after lap, goggles off, a full length with their heads underwater without taking a breath, goggles back on and then goggles off, another length without taking a breath, and so on for an hour. One day my son came out of the water in the middle of the first two sessions in tears, asking to go home.

'No,' I replied. 'Get back in the water. I am not taking you home until it is finished.'

As we drove past those same pools many years later, I overheard my son telling his friend of those horrible Sunday afternoons with the swim squad.

It was not until a friend told me that I needed to stop that I did. 'All you are doing is telling your son that you only appreciate and reward him when he does things that you value,' she said.

My son and I were incredibly close despite this. I still loved to jump into bed with him, although he probably did not love it so much. My mentor asked me one day if I ever hit him. She knew about my father and, more importantly, the acceptance of corporal punishment in Samoan society. But, in complete contrast to my father, I neither raised my voice nor struck my son, ever. Even with the strictest of fathers, I had always found a way to do what I wanted, and raising my child was no different. I preferred to raise my son free to do what he wanted, but also free to tell me about it.

* * *

One day in the middle of theatre, I received a call from my son's school. The anaesthetic technician picked it up and put it on speaker for me. 'Your son has fallen and he has back pain,' the school nurse reported.

'Can he walk?' I asked.

'Yes ...'

'Then give him some Panadol and send him back to class, please,' I replied. My operating list was on track to run over time, and I was stressed about the school calling me for something I felt they should have been able to manage.

After work, my son confronted me. I was flopped on the couch, and he was beside me, watching an episode of something on television. It was the end of a seven-day call week for me, and we had planned to have take-out and watch a movie, but I was exhausted. Catatonic. Unable to open my eyes. I nestled my head against him. It was still daylight outside.

'I think the school nurse was not happy with you today,' he said.

'I don't care,' I replied. 'The school nurse should be able to manage simple things like that. She wasted my time calling.'

'Your words become really hard when you have these busy weeks,' he told me. 'I don't like it, and it makes me anxious.'

I admired his assessment, and that he had mustered up the courage to say it. I think I managed to say sorry.

* * *

My mother's cancer recurred in less than two years. We saw it on a standard surveillance scan during one of her check-ups. The scan before that had been normal. Now, the recurrence was sitting where the old cancer had been, like it had just been hiding, waiting to reveal itself.

'I don't think this is surgically resectable,' the first surgeon said to us. Actually, he said it to me. My mother would defer to me in these appointments. I think she would have rather not been there.

'Okay,' I said co-operatively, mentally planning a list of every other surgeon I would consult.

I took her to multiple surgeons who I could imagine might re-operate to resect it, but the recurrence was a mass of lymph nodes, and we knew from the start that it had already spread through 35 of 35 lymph nodes as well as outside the lymph nodes. The recurrence was an inevitability. I asked a close friend who was also a highly skilled colorectal surgeon to operate. 'You can't do this, Ineke,' was the reply. 'We will achieve nothing.'

Damn.

I linked arms with my mother the day we walked out of her last surgeon's appointment. We were silent. Both afraid. 'One step at a time,' I told her. I had not even asked her if she wanted surgery.

On hearing the news, one colleague said bluntly, 'Well, at least the disease is retroperitoneal, and she will develop renal obstruction and fall into a coma. It could be worse.' He was right, and this is what I told myself because I was well familiar with the different patterns in which metastatic colon cancer manifested – but are we really so removed from humanity that this should have been interpreted as comforting?

She started back on chemotherapy. This was her new lifeline. She re-established herself in New Zealand, and we all silently accepted that she was in it for the long haul. I knew what that meant, but like most patients who encounter this hurdle she probably did not. It meant she would never be cured – she would die of her disease – and the chemotherapy might or might not help.

After returning from Sydney, where I had spent the year training as part of my breast-cancer and reconstruction specialisation, my son finally expressed how tired he was of moving all the time. So, he was enrolled into boarding school, and my mother lived at home with us, while I took a consultant job 100 kilometres south. We were like an exploded mini family bound together by necessity: my mother needed somewhere to live, and I needed her to help with my son while I worked.

In truth, I think she was happy to be living with me, and with her grandson. When I was young, I had always thought I would take my mother with me. I always knew that I would live far away from my family, but I thought I would take my mother with me. We had been incredibly close, and I had wanted to save her from her husband, but something had happened. Life probably. We were incapacitated by the years prior, my inability to understand her, and her unfulfilled desire for love and understanding from her eldest daughter.

One night, we decided to watch a movie at home. She had cooked dinner, as she did whenever she felt well enough. 'Here you go. Sit here.' She pointed to a comfortable part of the couch that she had vacated for me. It was right next to her.

'No, thanks. I will sit here,' I replied, walking past her and sitting on the part of the couch as far away as possible. I am sure I hurt her feelings that night, but I just could not be close to her, and I hated myself for it.

I was certainly a better doctor than a daughter. I still enjoyed the thrill of surgery, meeting people, making patients laugh, making sick patients better. Accompanying them. When I came home to my mother, however, I was stone cold. I had stopped her from asking medical questions of me at home, because I did not want to be her doctor, but I could not even be her daughter.

I often wondered how this was all going to end. I could not see in front of me. I could not see my future. I just had to keep all the balls in the air.

* * *

It had been a bizarre clinic on the day when a 19-year-old girl was referred for assessment because of a very large, very abnormal breast mass. I had already seen several ladies with very large advanced cancers, and I had the impression I was working in a Third World country, not a developed one with a national breast-screening programme.

This young girl was sitting in a consultation room alone, dressed in an oversized jersey covered by a big black puffer jacket. She looked glum, and sat with her shoulders hunched. In profile, she looked like a question mark. She had been 17 when her right breast exploded disproportionately in size relative to the left. There was no important family history of breast cancer and, apart from the disfiguring asymmetry, she was well. She did not have a boyfriend, and did not participate in any recreational activity because of the discrepancy, which meant she could not wear a supportive bra – or, indeed, anything other than that oversized jersey. More importantly, she was embarrassed. Mortified was the word she used.

It never fails to surprise me what people will tolerate. As a breast surgeon, I have seen a handful of women present with large, ulcerating breast cancers – one so large the woman had to cradle a mass the size of a football, and another who asked her pharmacist how she could mask the smell of rotting cancer on her chest wall. These women can go to work every day like this, and they can sleep with their husbands every night. Somehow, each day passes, and there is some acceptance of this new normal. This young girl had gone to her GP about another problem, and having identified this gross abnormality her doctor had appropriately referred her for imaging and assessment. The patient herself had not complained of the mass. The lump was the size of a large watermelon, which on a thin frame and in just the one breast, disfigured her completely. Fortunately, the lump was benign – juvenile fibroadenoma. But she needed it removed, and she needed her life back. How can people live like this for so long?

We spoke about surgery, the removal of the lump, the revision of the skin and how we would reshape the breast. She did not smile, she did not engage, but she signed the form for surgery.

The surgery itself was uncomplicated. The lump was removed, the skin and remaining breast reshaped, and I harvested fat from her hips using liposuction to fill some of the breast tissue that had been effaced by the huge watermelon that had been sitting against it for two years. I was happy with how she looked at the end of the case, although she still did not smile before she went home the next day.

It was not until her post-operative appointment some weeks later that I finally caught a glimpse of her teeth. This time she was with her mother, and this time she was happy. She told me she had not realised how bad she had looked until she went home after surgery and found she could look in the mirror again. She had already bought new bras. 'I should have had a goodbye party for my parasitic twin,' she said with a bright smile.

I did not expect the hug she gave me as she walked out the door, and I was moved by how much I had contributed to her newfound confidence.

* * *

In New Zealand, the national breast-screening programme offers free screening mammograms every two years for women aged between 45 and 69 years of age. Breast cancer is the most common cancer in women, with age being the biggest risk factor. Fortunately, because we have the ability to detect it early and cure it with standardised treatments, it is a cancer with established screening programmes in the developed world. Most breast cancers detected through the screening programme are in the early stages, slow-growing and small (in other words, you cannot feel them), and they are localised to the breast without having spread to the lymph nodes in the axilla.

At the age of 69, a lady presented with a low-grade, node-negative breast cancer. This woman, fortunately, had a 'good' type of cancer. People always look at us strangely when we say this, but there is a spectrum of possible outcomes depending on the breast cancer. By good, I mean that she had a 98 per cent chance of cure, as opposed to a woman with an aggressive breast-cancer subtype with multiple lymph nodes involved.

Our first consultation was for delivery of results. I told her that the mammogram and biopsy had unfortunately detected a small breast cancer, but this was very curable with surgery and radiotherapy. I reassured her that it had been caught early, that it had no adverse features, and that the treatment would be behind her in a matter of weeks.

She cried, which is very common and understandable, before she started to question what she had done in her life to deserve this. 'Why me?' she asked.

'It is nothing you've done. Unfortunately, the two biggest risk factors for breast cancer are being a woman and getting older,' I replied gently.

This seemed to appease her, and she left with a plan to return the following week to discuss surgery. The following week had evidently done her some good; she arrived at the clinic looking calm and well dressed, with her hair and make-up in order. These things are always good signs.

As I entered the consultation room, I closed the door behind me, and she pulled her phone from her bag. I told her she could ask her questions at the end, and insisted I examine her first. She was a little overweight, but otherwise in reasonable shape. She had large D-cup breasts with significant ptosis – this simply means that the breasts have drooped with age, breastfeeding and gravity. They can droop a little, or they can droop a lot. Unfortunately, we cannot fight it. I finished my examination and, when she was dressed, we sat down face to face to speak about her operation.

'I want to show you something,' she said frankly. On her phone, she showed me a photo of a young, tall 20-something woman with caramel skin and full-projection breast implants. She was wearing a skimpy white bikini, and probably holidaying in Miami – or, as we have come to learn of the extremes that influencers will go to, just lying in her backyard on a mountain of sand.

'What's this?' I asked her.

'I've been doing lots of research over the last week, and I've decided that I want you to make my breasts better at the same time as my cancer operation. Make them tight and high. Like this girl. Tight and high,' she repeated.

I remembered a hairdresser once telling me that his pet peeve was clients bringing in photos of celebrities, asking for a haircut like Jessica Alba's. (Okay, I am guilty of that one.) He recounted a client bringing in a photo of Khloé Kardashian, and requesting to look exactly like her. He told his client that he could duplicate her hairstyle, but he could never make her look like Khloé.

Me? With this woman, I kept quiet and counted to ten before opening my mouth. A consultant I worked for years ago once told me I should do this.

It is even more amusing – and by this, I mean it is not – when we are asked by spouses for 'tight and high'. Not infrequently, I have been asked by a husband if I can make his wife's breasts bigger when we are talking about reconstruction after breast cancer. And, several times, husbands have asked for an 'extra stitch' to tighten a post-birth vaginal canal when I have managed their wives' haemorrhoids. It is another count-to-ten situation. Maybe 20.

* * *

Body dysmorphic disorder (BDD) is a preoccupation with an imagined anomaly in one's appearance, or an excessive preoccupation with a minor flaw. For the affected person, it can be incredibly distressing and may be linked to previous trauma, so it should never be minimalised. Imagine how you might feel with a pimple on your nose – it might be all that you see in the mirror, but it could be that no one else sees it. This is how BDD feels.

A young man in his twenties made an appointment to see me about a nipple reduction. The referral letter said it was causing him much distress – he was unable to go to the gym and was ashamed in the dressing rooms. But he was a busy young man, and we had to reschedule his appointment several times. Finally, he asked if I would see him on the weekend or after hours, because he was coming from out of town and his work hours precluded him from getting there on my clinic days. I agreed, as this was obviously causing him distress. He was fit and young, and clearly very anxious. He hated his nipples, he told me. They were big and he wanted them reduced. They were visible through his T-shirt, and they were swollen. I listened to his concerns and noted them down.

We talked about his general health, what he did for work and if he lived with family. Did he have a lover? What did his nipples stop him from doing? When I had sufficiently filled in all the boxes to paint a picture of his general life and his functional impairment, I asked him to take off his top so that I could examine him. My eyes met two perfectly normal and symmetrical nipples. I held my tongue for a few seconds as I carefully calculated my response. 'Point out exactly what bothers you,' I said.

He pinched and pulled at his nipples, to show me how excessive and prominent they were, and I nodded slowly as I listened. When he had finished explaining the source of his distress, I told him I thought his nipples were perfectly normal, and that with any surgical intervention we risked wound problems and scarring, asymmetry and, more importantly, making things worse for him. He persevered over this, clarifying and re-clarifying his concerns and my answers. It seemed we were doomed to ruminate in circles – until he asked for the cost of surgery. After that, he promptly informed me that he would need time to think and left.

Two others that week had exited in the same fashion. A young woman had demanded to have fat put in her lower back, where she thought there was a dent. I could not see the dent, even though we went to the mirror and I asked her to point out exactly where the dent was. 'To be honest, I cannot appreciate a dent. Everything looks completely normal to me,' I responded slowly.

Another young man saw me because he wanted a rib removed. He was certain it was sticking out.

The alarm bell is always when you see that you are the fourth surgeon that a patient has visited. An important part of being a good surgeon is knowing when not to operate, and when to call for help. I now have a cognitive behavioural therapist in my phonebook.

* * *

There are certain subspecialties within surgery that require substantial input from psychologists, who help us improve patient outcomes, experiences and expectations. Managing expectations is an important part of surgery, and in certain subspecialties where people are transforming their bodies and lives it is vital. One example is patients who are about to embark on weight-loss surgery, and although it is less routine I am convinced it should also include women undergoing breast reconstruction after cancer. I was even more convinced of this after one particular Tuesday morning.

Given it was my subspecialty, 50 per cent of my practice was breast-cancer surgery and reconstruction. For me, Tuesday mornings were usually a busy breast clinic in which I would see new cancers, have follow-ups with patients who'd had surgery in previous weeks, and see long-standing patients undergoing breast reconstruction. As I sat in my office, reading and preparing the next file for a new breast-cancer diagnosis, my registrar walked in looking flustered. It seemed the patient she was seeing was not happy with her breast reconstruction. The registrar was at a loss, because her objective assessment by all measures was that the reconstruction was exceptionally good.

Breast reconstruction can be a challenging practice. Social media and certain high-profile celebrities who have undergone major surgery for breast cancer and breast-cancer risk have somehow created the impression that reconstructive surgery is synonymous with cosmetic surgery, and that it is an opportunity to have better breasts. While the goal is always to reconstruct a breast that looks as normal as possible after removing it because of cancer, to achieve a perfectly identical match with the other side is challenging, and not infrequently impossible. In addition to this, reconstruction is never complete after one operation; often it takes several procedures to get right.

In this case, however, I had to agree with my registrar. This particular woman looked great. She was well matched for size. The shape was superb, and the cleavage was perfect. She even had the classic tan lines to show how proud she was of her décolletage. It's a classic before-and-after for those who attend plastic-surgical meetings. Before picture: a pale woman with small breasts and no tan lines. After picture: the same woman, now buxom, with tan lines indicating a string bikini and lots of sun. Tan lines are always a good sign that a woman is proud enough of her new cleavage to parade it on a public beach. And this lady had these exact tan lines.

'What are you unhappy with?' I asked, feeling tension rise in my shoulders. It was not lost on me that this lady had undergone four revision procedures and always found something new to be dissatisfied with.

She got down on her hands and knees, in a position I didn't imagine her to actually be in very often (some might call it doggy style), then pushed her reconstructed breast in with one hand. 'When I am in this position, can you see the slight flattening on the top here when I push the breast this way?'

My silence conveyed how unimpressed I was.

'Sometimes, the light catches it, and then you can really see it. I just don't think the light is in the right place now,' she added to justify herself, while continuing to try to simulate the exact position on her hands and knees in which this subtle flattening could apparently be seen.

Another woman, who was in her late fifties, presented for consideration of a delayed chest-wall reconstruction. She'd had a mastectomy about five years prior for breast cancer, and had been given the all-clear the year before. She wanted to return to normal, and was considering her options for reconstruction. By the time she came to see me, I was her fourth opinion – as I've said, always a sign. She had consulted two local plastic surgeons, and had even travelled to the United States for another opinion. Upon recommendation from another, she made an appointment to attend my clinic.

She was in great shape. Successful in her career, very fit, good form. She had several options for reconstruction, but as is usually the case there was a stand-out option. We discussed in great detail each option, the pros and cons, and I pulled open my laptop to show her what she might realistically look like with each type of reconstruction. We spent about 45 minutes in the first consultation, then I offered her a second appointment to discuss her thoughts and any questions that might have developed in the interim. When she attended this second appointment, she was still in massive doubt, which meant that there was absolutely no urgency on my part to do anything. I really wanted her to go away and think carefully, and perhaps speak with another specialist or other patients. Reconstruction is a tough journey, and both patient and surgeon need to be in it 100 per cent.

She sat quietly for a moment before she voiced her thoughts. 'I just need a surgeon who can understand how personal this is for me. It's not heart surgery. It's reconstruction of my breast. It's very personal.'

I was taken aback by her comparison. 'I'm sure that every woman and man who has had heart surgery thought it was pretty personal to have their heart opened by someone they have known for less than a month,' I replied.

Exasperation is really what I felt at the end of such clinics. They were overbooked, with women waiting one to two hours on occasion. There was not enough operating space for us to deal with first diagnoses of cancer, let alone a fourth or fifth reconstruction revision. Women were not happy about having to wait, reception staff and nurses (except for the brilliant twosome who worked with me – they were amazing) were not happy because patients were complaining, booking clerks were not happy because there were no operating lists to put patients into, and I was just trying to get through the morning.

* * *

I am sure AJ thought she saw too much of me. She was back and forth for at least two years because of me. Her breast cancer was detected through a routine screening mammogram, but nothing was straightforward.

Initially, she had a single focus of breast cancer, which on the day of her surgery had increased to five foci. That was a surprise. I tried to salvage her breast with a fancy conservation procedure, meaning that I resected the five foci of cancer en bloc, and then reshaped the remaining breast tissue so that the excision did not leave her breast deformed. Unfortunately, the specimen showed cancer extending to its edges under the microscope, meaning the excision was incomplete.

With five spots of cancer, it probably was not so much of a surprise that this was the case, but in a woman who has the possibility of keeping her breast and is motivated to do so I will always give lumpectomy (or lumpectomies, as it was in this case) a chance, as long as she understands that there is a reasonable risk of a second operation. AJ also had positive lymph nodes. She needed chemotherapy and radiotherapy. And a mastectomy.

We decided to keep her options open for reconstruction, and she went forward for six months of chemotherapy first, followed by three weeks of radiotherapy. On her chemotherapy regime, she gained over ten kilograms, which makes any cancer surgeon's heart sink. Reconstruction would be difficult. Nonetheless, AJ was always bright. She smiled and spoke and laughed voraciously, and she had a formidable ally in her husband. I witnessed this alliance after her first operation. They came to clinic with her drain chart, which her husband had been keeping so devotedly that, while she slept, he would lie awake by her bed watching the drains, documenting their outputs and making sure they were still working. I certainly had the impression that all three of us were on this path together.

AJ required a tissue reconstruction, but her only option was for tissue transfer from her back to her chest wall. Implant reconstruction would not suit her shape, and her weight exceeded the recommendation for tissue transfer from the abdominal wall. We spoke at length about this type of reconstruction during her chemotherapy, and then before and after radiotherapy.

The day for her surgery arrived and, although challenging, the surgery itself was uncomplicated, and she went home three days later. I was proud of myself for persevering through surgery when many would have declined reconstruction based on her weight. But as a surgeon, you quickly learn not to count your chickens. You can never be truly certain that you are in the clear until weeks after surgery.

Unfortunately, within a week AJ's skin had started to blister, and within two weeks the skin over her lower breast had peeled completely, leaving a large area of raw tissue underneath. This was surprise number three. She required daily nursing visits to apply specialised dressings to the reconstruction for weeks on end.

Weeks turned into months and finally the skin was healed, and this first part was over. She then required more surgery to finish the reconstruction. Further operative procedures over the following months included fat-grafting to the reconstruction to improve its aesthetic appearance, and then finally a small breast reduction on the other side so that she would be more symmetrical. It was a very long path, and I could see at times that, as brave and bubbly as she was, AJ was also tired.

Some months after it was all done, AJ spoke at a charity event and chronicled her path. She told her audience that only that morning she had looked in the mirror and felt normal again for the first time in over 12 months.

I always tell my patients embarking on breast reconstruction that it is a long path, with multiple operations, but often this is still not enough to prepare them. It requires mental fortitude and commitment from both parties, and it really is a journey.

For AJ, more than two years after endless hospital visits, chemotherapy, radiotherapy, and multiple surgeries, she was cancer-free, and she could confidently look at herself in the mirror, happy with the long path we had all decided to take together.

* * *

At the age of 30, KB had discovered a lump in her right breast. In fact, it was her partner who had found the lump, as is often the case in this age group. She had seen her GP, who also felt the lump and initiated investigation. A mammogram and ultrasound showed that this lump was almost certainly cancerous, and a needle biopsy confirmed it was what we call triple-positive breast cancer.

Breast cancer might be the most commonly diagnosed cancer among women, but at the age of 30 it is not at all common and represents a mere 1 per cent of all diagnosed breast cancers. When we look at a cancer under the microscope, we look at a number of things that help us to determine how aggressive it is, and therefore whether or not it will benefit from certain treatments, such as chemotherapy or other targeted drugs. The more aggressive a breast cancer is, or the more adverse features that exist, the greater the benefit chemotherapy will provide. Under the microscope, KB's cancer had all the hallmarks of aggressive disease. It was grade three, meaning that the cells were deformed and no longer resembled anything close to normal, and it expressed oestrogen, progesterone and the HER2 receptor.

All breast cancers are tested for these three receptors. Approximately 80 per cent of breast cancers are oestrogen- and/or progesterone-receptor positive, which means that the cancer responds to circulating oestrogen and/ or progesterone. This is important, because blocking or manipulating oestrogen and progesterone in the body after surgery, chemotherapy or radiotherapy can reduce the risk of cancer coming back in the breast (or elsewhere in the body), and reduce the chance of a new cancer in the other breast. It can also ultimately maximise the chance of cure.

As well as telling us that she was oestrogen and progesterone positive, KB's biopsy also told us that she was HER2 positive. In the early 1980s, when HER2 was first discovered, this meant aggressive and rapid growth, and a survival in years measured on one hand. In the late 1990s, however, Herceptin, a therapy targeted at blocking HER2 expression, revolutionised the treatment of women with HER2-positive disease, reduced recurrence rates and improved overall survival.

Immediately after her diagnosis, KB had undergone surgery: a standard lumpectomy, and removal of all the lymph nodes in her axilla, because the cancer cells had already spread to the lymph nodes in her armpit. Unfortunately, the lumpectomy was not successful. Under the pathologist's microscopic lens, it was found that the cancer was invading blood vessels throughout the breast tissue that had been removed, and cancer was found extending to every edge of the excised specimen. This meant that her cancer had not been completely removed with the lumpectomy. She required chemotherapy and Herceptin as a priority, to be followed by removal of the rest of her breast (mastectomy), and then radiotherapy. Chemotherapy would be given for six months – an intravenous infusion every three weeks for the first three months, and then weekly for the second three months. And yes, she would lose her hair. The Herceptin would be given for 12 months.

Losing her hair is not the only aspect a 30-year-old woman worries about. KB was in the prime of her working life. She and her partner were engaged, and had planned to get married that year, then to start a family shortly after. Chemotherapy can have a huge impact on a young woman's fertility, because of the nature of the drugs. The desired effect is to kill the most rapidly dividing cells in the body – and, for a woman in her reproductive years, this includes the cells in her ovaries. Moreover, a woman might be at her peak fertility and want to have a family, but she must put all this on hold for years while she completes treatment.

It is for this reason that we offer women in a reproductive age group the chance of fertility preservation before they start their systemic treatment. With breast cancer, this includes cryopreservation of embryos or oocyte (egg) cryopreservation. Other cancers might require additional protections, such as repositioning the ovaries, and this depends on the requirements for treatment. KB wanted to utilise the option of embryo preservation, as she had the future father of her children in her fiancé. Some women don't have the option of storing embryos, and therefore can only store eggs. So, with the help of a fertility specialist, two embryos were put on ice, to be used after KB got through all of her treatment.

I didn't meet KB and her fiancé until a year after her diagnosis, once her chemotherapy was complete. She needed a mastectomy, and wanted breast reconstruction with it. I was impressed with their cool factor from the moment I met them. KB was petite with flawless skin and perfectly applied black wing-tipped eyeliner that I would forever admire because I lacked the skill to apply it as she did, and she wore beautiful headscarves. And her fiancé, nonchalant but not really, dressed in black, always.

KB had come through her chemotherapy well, and we decided that she would go forward for a mastectomy with immediate reconstruction using an implant. The decision-making, of course, was not so simple. KB was trying to get through her treatment, wanted a romantic island wedding, wanted to breastfeed her children, and wanted to never have to go through breast cancer again. She wanted to survive. Fair enough for a woman of 30. We spoke about all these things.

In total, she had ten centimetres of grade-three breast cancer, with eight lymph nodes that were positive. This is what we would call locally advanced. We have clever applications and statistical programmes that can spit out a patient's chances of survival using age, the grade of cancer, the receptors it expresses, how big it is and the number of nodes involved. When we entered KB's data, the programme told us that, of 100 women with the exact features of her disease, only seven would be alive ten years after surgery, chemotherapy and Herceptin. But here's the thing about numbers: we did not know where KB fell on that line. She could be one of the seven. And she sure lived like it.

I reconstructed KB, and performed two further revision surgeries to complete the reconstruction. Over that time, she ran away to the islands and got married, her hair grew back, and she returned to work full-time (she never stopped working). When I last saw her, she was five weeks pregnant with one of her embryos.

Bravo, KB. As we say in New Zealand, legend.

I was so proud of her, and so proud to know her.

10.

Everything that matters hurts

My mother was dependent on chemotherapy.

'How long does this go on for?' she asked me one day as we were folding the washing together. Our lives had taken on a more established routine. She had always loved to keep a home and make food for her children, and this is what she was doing for us in between feeling rotten from chemotherapy. I was flying or driving up and down the country for work, and returning home to her and my son when I could do so in the weekends.

'When you decide you have had enough,' I replied.

'How do I decide?'

'When, one day, you wake up here, stuck to chemotherapy, and you feel like you are not living your life, and that you would rather be in Samoa, free, in your garden, underneath the sun, surrounded by your sisters, brothers and children,' I replied.

She stayed on chemotherapy for the better part of a year, and in that time she would request treatment breaks to go back to Samoa. Her heart was there. She had a beautiful, lush garden at home, and she missed the contact with her own family. She was isolated in New Zealand, living through her cycles of chemotherapy, wondering if she would ever get back to a 'normal' life.

Each treatment break was only a matter of weeks, but with each she had evidence of disease progression on repeat scanning, which meant that she really required the chemotherapy to stay alive. Furthermore, her trips back to Samoa were causing tension between us, because she was returning to her home, where my father still lived. He was not well. Time had not been kind, and he was increasingly disinhibited and paranoid, which meant that, when she was home, my mother could not be left alone with him. He was still reasonably independent, but he was behaving erratically, and required some supervision to ensure he was eating normally and paying attention to his daily cares.

We all loved our mother, and so without hesitation someone was always there to protect her and ensure that my father would leave her in peace. Sometimes, she would lock herself in her room for privacy, and he would bang at the door, wanting to get inside. He would not stop. More precisely, he *could* not stop, because his brain injury had impacted his ability to think. My sister would not leave my mother's side to intervene and redirect him.

I was angry at my mother for always going back to a situation that she knew would end badly, and for putting her children in those situations. I was angry that debt was pouring out of every orifice, and that my siblings were discussing how to manage it, which was affecting their own lives and their ability to build new ones. I was angry that they had not done better. For my own selfishness, I decided that I could not take part in any debt repayments, which seemed to be at least six figures, endless and unsustainable. 'Just let everything fall,' I said to my sister on the phone one evening.

'I want to do this for Mum.' She was dutiful. 'I found her crying today,' she continued. 'Dad just hounds her relentlessly. He is accusing her of cheating on him.'

I sighed. Fuck. Why? 'Yes, but he is not well and we know this!' I replied. 'The only one who can change this situation is her. She has to remove herself.'

Of course, she should have been free to live peacefully in her home, which she loved, but the situation was untenable. The whole drama was getting in the way of what should have been a peaceful time for everyone, especially for her.

When she returned to New Zealand, her scan again showed some progression, and she recommended chemotherapy, but after a couple of months I noticed that she was not the same. She was tired, and she was in pain. One day, I found her crying in her room, unable to find relief from the unrelenting back pain. I took her to the hospital so that she could have the pain relief she needed, and we waited for another scan.

Her sisters flew in from around New Zealand and across the Tasman Sea to be with her. They stayed with her when, two days later, the oncologist told her there was nothing more to do. That the cancer had escaped and had done so rapidly. They were there when the oncologist said she would not see Christmas. Me? I was in a staff meeting that I could not cancel. At least she was with her sisters. They had coffee in a park nearby, and cried underneath a cruel sun.

It was September. The oncologist sent me the images, so that I could see them from my breast clinic. I had seen images like it many times before, but when it is your own mother you can hardly believe it.

I arrived home that night to find my mother and her sisters lying in her room. They were talking and laughing, and one of her sisters was lying against her in bed, holding her and massaging her back. I felt guilty for not having been able to lie against my mother like that, for not comforting her in a soft or loving way, for not comforting her in the way that she had needed. I really wished that I could have, but our relationship had changed. I did not feel light. Our walls of silence over the last five years, maybe more, just stood there between us. Dense. We had moved around each other in circles, in silence, just trying to make things work.

She had decided to return to Samoa within days. One of her sisters would accompany her on the flight. We busied ourselves getting prescriptions filled for pain relief and any other symptom we could possibly imagine. There was no possibility that she would be able to find what she needed reliably in Samoa, so we had to prepare.

I was realising that my mother would leave and never return to New Zealand, where we had spent so much time together. On the night before she was due to fly, I found her lying in her bedroom, alone. I climbed into bed with her, no longer able to control my tears. I had spent many nights crying over our 'situation', but I had not cried at the idea of losing my mother. My heart was broken. The last time I had jumped into bed with her had probably been when I was eight years old.

'I don't want you to go,' I whispered, as I sobbed uncontrollably. I was lying on my back against her, tears streaming down my face. She put her arm around me and cried silently also. 'You must be tired,' I said. 'You never deserved this.'

We descended into sadness, lost in our thoughts again, unsure of how to start, unsure if we could say everything we wanted to.

'You are my firstborn,' she finally said. 'And I have been so happy to be your mother. I remember when you took your first step, and it was the happiest moment of my life. I am proud of you.'

We spoke of the past, of the years long before then. How she had been so happy raising her family. How she had been so sad losing her own mother. We did not speak of my father, or of the years prior when all there had been to talk about was illness and money. The road had been hard, and at the age of 59 years, she wanted to make it to her sixtieth birthday a month later in October, and to Christmas day, and she wanted to see the birth of her grandchild in the New Year.

'I will always be with you,' she told me. 'When the clouds part, and the sun shines through them, that will be me.'

I cried and cried against her, and when it was midnight I kissed her goodbye, and went to pack for my week. I had to leave at 5 a.m. the next morning to be the acute surgeon on call for the weekend.

* * *

When my mother returned to Samoa to die, her siblings dropped everything to be by her side. Every day they sat with her, held her, massaged her and prayed with her.

My own siblings surprised me. My youngest sister, who was training to be a physiotherapist, finished the year early, and slept alongside our mother, waking every morning to massage her swollen leg and carrying her to the shower when she finally became immobile. Every one of the others took their turn to comfort and hold our mother. They were all amazing.

From the moment that I had left home 20 years prior, I had not wanted to go back. But now I returned, and only because it was necessary. I had wanted as little as possible to do with family, but now I finally felt lucky to be part of this tribe. It was my mother's tribe. It was strange to be among this. It was even stranger that I loved to be a part of it again. I spent the next ten weeks flying back and forth as much as possible around work, my son in tow, to spend time with her.

My mother was constantly surrounded by family, and by early December we had moved a hospital bed into her room to make it easier for transferring her and changing her position. She mustered enough energy to oversee the Christmas tree being cut down in the backyard and erected on the porch, but the week before Christmas her pain was escalating and she was sleepy. We knew she was dying. I had already asked a doctor at the national hospital for morphine that I could administer to keep her comfortable. There was no such thing as palliative care in Samoa. We would have to take care of it.

On Christmas Eve, my mother asked me if we could go for a ride to get ice cream. She was almost immobile, and suffering severe pain and limb swelling due to her pelvic lymph nodes. I could see it when I helped her to change. But that evening, my sisters and I lifted her into the car, and the two of us drove for ice cream, just as we had done 30 years prior when she had learnt to drive. We said nothing. We ate our ice cream in silence. Those trips for ice cream had been our thing. Our getaway from the house when I was seven years old.

The next morning, Christmas, I woke to find her crying in bed. I did not understand why, and she did not say. My father sat next to her, unsure, I think. We were not paying attention to him. We all sat around her bed, trying to feign happiness – opening presents, saying thank you, watching her. Her eyes were vacant, and we knew we were losing her. My sisters hid their faces from her as they cried at the head of her bed. I grabbed her hand and told her that I would miss her and that I loved her.

We carried her into her garden, bathed in the sunlight of Christmas Day, and she pointed out where she wanted to be buried: underneath one of her favourite trees. She thanked us for everything we had done, and then, sitting in her wheelchair overlooking the garden where she had escaped to find peace most days, she slipped into unconsciousness. She remained in a coma for four days before she finally died.

* * *

Mr H bowled me over with his bravery. He was 35 years old – two years younger than me when I had been the general surgeon on call, and the same age as my resident, whose voice broke, choked by tears, when he told me about Mr H. 'I'm sorry,' he said, apologising for the falter. 'It's just too close to home.'

Not only were the resident and Mr H the same age, but they had both recently welcomed their firstborns into the world. Mr H had been abroad with his beautiful wife and a 12-month-old, but he had not been well for some months, with various aches and pains, which he had ignored. Now that he was home, things were worse than ever. He came to hospital because his left eye was not moving properly, and he was seeing double. He also complained of abdominal pain, bloating and feeling full after small meals. He had lost a lot of weight as a result.

A scan revealed everything we hate to see: a large colon cancer on the right, multiple enlarged lymph nodes along blood vessels supplying the colon, multiple spots of cancer in the lungs, multiple spots of cancer along the abdominal wall. As my resident scrolled down the scan, I felt as if my own insides were being squeezed. It was the same sensation I'd had when I'd opened my mother's scan, confronted by the disease and the knowledge that nothing more could be done after years of chemotherapy.

In most cancer units, a weekly multidisciplinary meeting convenes to ensure best practice for all new cancer diagnoses, and for any challenging cases. It is where surgeons, medical and radiation oncologists, radiologists, pathologists, physicians, specialist nurses, radiographers and cancer co-ordinators sit, listen to a clinical history, review imaging and inspect pathology results. It is where dispositions and optimal treatment sequences are discussed, and treatment plans documented.

For people such as Mr H – with his story, his scans and his blood tests – there is always a palpable heaviness in the room. The silence, the delayed breaths, the sadness knowing what the future holds. It hits the same every time, and with Mr H it was worse. He was young, he had a new baby, and he had months that you could count on one hand left to live. His only chance was chemotherapy, and even then, with the disease peppered throughout his body, there was no cure. Chemotherapy would only afford him more time. Without it, he was looking at a survival of about three months.

He had a large right-sided colon cancer partially obstructing the lumen, and we were worried he was going to run into trouble with a complete blockage or perforation during chemotherapy, so a plan was made to operate and remove this urgently. It was at this point that I met Mr H and his wife, as I was the surgeon on call. After introducing myself to both of them, we spoke about his story. I reiterated his scan findings, and then I examined his abdomen. I recall feeling firmness over his general abdomen – a little more firmness than I would have expected for the large colon cancer we had seen on his scan. Before taking him through to theatre, I obtained his consent, and he asked whether there was a chance that I would open him, find him inoperable and close him again.

'There is a chance that the scan has underestimated your disease, and that I might not be able to remove the colon cancer,' I told him honestly. 'But I will do my very best so that you can begin chemotherapy as quickly as possible.'

It was a difficult and sad moment, because I could only imagine his fear, and the last thing I wanted was for him to go to sleep feeling anxious, scared and hopeless.

With Mr H's abdomen open, everything told me there was no way I could do anything safely for him. He had a huge conglomerate mass of lymph nodes running along all his major blood vessels to his intestines, extending up and down and right and left. I gasped as I ran my hands over the mass, hating the way this disease consumed once-healthy bodies, hating what I knew was in store for him. The mass was solid and rough and gross, and lymphatic fluid bathed his bowels because the cancer had stopped the normal circulation.

I called a colleague whose subspecialty was colon cancer, to see if he could offer anything I was failing to see. We pontificated over a huge resection, intestinal bypasses, stomas ... but we both knew that anything we did would make him worse, significantly delay his recovery and perhaps truly impair the ability for him to have chemotherapy safely. 'Sorry, mate,' my colleague whispered, as we closed Mr H. Two fully qualified surgeons are not necessary to suture skin, but my colleague did not leave me. We were united by sadness for this young man who was so much like us.

I called Mr H's wife to tell her we had closed, then I waited for him to wake up.

Imagine a young man thanking you for trying when you tell him there was nothing you could do. He smiles and tells you it is okay. And, while you are fighting tears, he is trying to comfort you. Every morning I saw Mr H, he smiled the same smile, as he renewed his focus on a trial of chemotherapy, which would hopefully give him more time with his wife and baby. He spent two weeks in hospital, ensuring that the commencement of chemotherapy was safe so early after surgery.

'I wish you the very best,' I told him on the last morning before he was discharged. 'You are so brave and I admire you so much.'

I was there with my team, and he was smiling as he did every day. There was a dense silence in the room. No more words. Eyes wet with tears. It was unlikely our paths would ever cross again.

* * *

Mrs S was 31 years old when she first found a lump in her right breast, and 11 weeks pregnant. For at least a year, she and her husband had been trying to conceive, and now they were just one week away from the end of the first trimester – a date at which they had decided their wonderful news would be shared with their families.

Unfortunately, the ultrasound of her breast looked suspicious, and a biopsy confirmed the worst. It was a grade-three breast cancer, and she needed surgery, chemotherapy and radiotherapy. It is a classic case for our consultancy exams: a young woman who is 11 weeks pregnant presents with an aggressive breast cancer. What would you do?

We spoke at length with Mrs S about her treatment options, and the possibilities of sequencing her treatment. She was going to require chemotherapy, and we know chemotherapy is safe to administer to a woman in her second trimester, which she would be within days. We recommended that she undergo surgery immediately for the breast cancer, then start chemotherapy when she had recovered in a few weeks' time.

It is easy for us to give information. We have given it many times before. But, if we see 20 different patients, we must give it 20 different ways. After an hour-long conversation, Mrs S and her husband were in shock. They were young, newly married and had just moved to another country to start a new life. They were devastated. A million questions and just as many answers, and sometimes the same questions and answers. This is grief. They were worried about their new baby – the short-term implications of toxic treatment, and the long-term expectations for a new mother's life. Would the chemotherapy kill their baby? And if not, would Mrs S survive the disease to see her baby grow? With what we knew, her chance of being alive ten years after surgery and chemotherapy was 75 per cent. Fantastic odds. But people interpret numbers in different ways. The conversations were long and emotional, and much time was spent between the breast surgeon, the medical oncologist and the obstetrician.

On the day of her breast surgery, Mrs S arrived in the operating bay with her eyes red and swollen from two weeks of tears. She broke down as she explained that they had decided to terminate the pregnancy once her breast had been removed. She sobbed as she told us that she could not bear the possibility that her child might grow up without a mother. For her, the 25 per cent risk that she would not be around for her ten-year-old child was too much.

Through our own tears, we stayed by her side as she went to sleep, each of us heavy with thoughts of our own mortality. Each of us conscious of the fact that it could have been any one of us on that table considering a life in which we might not see our own children grow.

* * *

JC was just 26 when her brother wrapped her in a blanket, put her on a plane and held her every moment of their four-hour flight to New Zealand. He told her to act normal so she wouldn't alert airline staff. He was trying to save her life.

A year earlier, she'd had surgery in her home country, a developing nation in the South Pacific, for an advanced cancer of the rectum, but because chemotherapy and radiotherapy – standard treatments in rectal cancer – are not available in most Pacific nations, it had recurred very early. In truth, a 25-year-old should not have a rectal cancer, and it is logical that the biology of this disease in someone far too young is never good. Such was the case for JC. The very aggressive recurrence had terrible consequences: she could not eat or drink, and her intestinal content was no longer travelling through her intestinal tract. Instead, it was exiting to her abdominal wall in multiple places where the cancer had blocked normal passage and formed abnormal connections with the skin over the abdominal wall. Each one of these abnormal exits from the gut to the skin is called a fistula.

The two main problems this presented were severe and overwhelming infection, and malnutrition. JC had undergone emergency surgery in her home country several weeks earlier, but it had not been successful. After a two-week stay in the public hospital, her family had been told to take her home to die. Refusing to believe that this was the end, they had tried to get financial aid from the government to get her to New Zealand, but this had been futile. So they had taken out a loan to buy two airline tickets, she said goodbye to her husband and four young children, and she boarded the plane with her brother. The plane was her lifeboat.

When she arrived at hospital, she was severely malnourished. She was emaciated, her eyes too big for her face, her ribcage protruding sharply through her skin, and two large bags over her abdominal wall were full of faecal content that was much too watery. Her brother's eyes were tired and sad. He was her guardian, and spent nearly every moment on the floor by her bedside, emptying the effluent as it filled the bags adhering to the excoriated skin beneath her oversized T-shirts. There was nothing we could do for her surgically and, with the malnutrition, even feeding her intravenously was not going to save her. The disease had consumed – *was* consuming – her body, and she was dying. She nodded and smiled as I told her that this really was the end of the road for her. We expected her to live for a period of days to weeks. Not even a month.

Now the emergency was to organise visas for her husband and children, find money for five airline tickets and fly her family to New Zealand to say goodbye. With the hospital support staff, expert at managing difficult situations, visas and airline tickets were acquired, and within two weeks her family members were on their way over.

My heart hurt every morning that I went to see JC and her brother. For this reason, she had to be the last patient on the ward round, because we simply could not see another after her. At the age of 26, she was on borrowed time. She was grateful for the care she was receiving – she told us so every morning – and she was relieved to have taken the chance to get to us, even though fate had different plans for her.

I cried every morning that I visited her, and when she was finally transferred to the hospice for her last days my heart broke. I cried every day that I saw her in the hospice, and when her mother, her husband and her young children finally arrived to say goodbye I did not go back. When she died, I was ashamedly relieved, because I could no longer bear the sadness. After her death, the hospice staff said she was disappointed that I did not go back because she had wanted her mother to meet me.

11.

Teach me to feel another's woe

I have heard many a patient say that they leave their dignity at the door when they come into the hospital. This is usually in reference to having a breast examination or a rectal examination. But what can be said for those who do not have the capacity to make a conscious decision to leave their dignity, or relinquish their autonomy, wherever and whenever they choose?

I was on call and surrounded by the typical buzz of activity in the emergency department. Our team had descended on the doctors' write-up, a large central area surrounded by cubicles – resuscitation at one end, ambulatory at the other, and occupied trollies in hallways every which way you looked – to assess a new referral. The patient was an elderly woman with dementia. She had been brought in from her rest home at an ungodly hour perhaps because she had winced when the nursing staff touched her abdomen, or maybe she had vomited. Often the story is unclear. These patients are difficult to assess, and often the corroborating history is poor because they cannot tell us their version of events. The sad truth is, no one can.

She had been parked in one of the smaller cubicles next to the ambulatory assessment area – ambulatory meaning that people are walking, and their visits are expected to be quick, usually a sprained ankle or a broken finger after evening sport. But she was not walking, her visit was definitely not going to be quick, and her problems were not easily fixable. The nurses had kindly turned off her cubicle light to lull her into a restful slumber amid the endless activity and the front desk's frequent announcements of various triage categories.

We crept into the room and opened the curtain slightly to allow the light from the main area to illuminate her temporary abode, hoping it would be easy to examine her. I secretly hoped she was fast asleep and that we would not even wake her. If patients are not co-operative, then assessment of their abdomen is impossible, as they tense or strain against the touch and pressure of a total stranger. Understandable. But what struck me as I entered the cubicle was the smell. It was putrid – absolutely horrible. I gagged, opened the curtains fully and turned on the light to find the walls and bedside rails completely smeared with brown stools. Her right hand was the nail in the coffin.

I was aghast, thinking that it was pretty disgusting for somebody to do such a thing. I was soon to learn my lesson for passing such a judgement.

* * *

After my mother's death, it became apparent that, in being so consumed by her illness, we had all missed our father's decline. By the time we noticed, he was on a path of rapid deterioration, with zero capacity to safely care for himself. My sister called me one day. 'We found Dad on the floor this morning,' she said. 'He could not get himself up, and he is confused.'

Fearing a stroke, I asked her to put him on the plane. Various tests in the hospital confirmed that it was a urine infection, and he was appropriately given antibiotics and flew back to Samoa.

Within a month, he was on the plane again. He had been doing strange things like putting cereal over the top of his rice at dinner, but it was another fall that brought him back. This time, he required an extended stay in the hospital. His objective assessments, such as the mini mental-state exam, which measures cognitive function, were significantly worse than when he had been in hospital just over a month prior. At the age of 62, he was diagnosed with advanced dementia. He required hospital-level care because the simple act of dressing or showering – something so many of us take for granted – was too confusing for him, and he also required constant supervision. The circle of life is real.

He had two options: he could return to Samoa, and we could find help to care for him, but the facilities for dementia were not well established there, or he could stay in New Zealand and be placed in a dementia unit here. We were overcome with sadness again, anguished over which option would be best for him. We decided that his access to medical care and organised activities for patients with dementia was the highest priority, so he stayed in New Zealand.

The moment that I walked into his new home, I started to cry. Never had I imagined that my father would end up in a dementia unit at the age of 62. He was far too young, still physically fit, walking down the hallway saying 'Hello, mate' to everyone he passed. He did not fit in with the 80-year-old lady holding onto her doll and plastered to an armchair in the TV room, or with the man across the hall who was bedbound, gazing into the heavens, while his private TV blasted Coca-Cola advertisements. I wiped my eyes, and feigned a smile so that my father would not see my distress. He, however, could not hide his. 'Get me out of here,' he said through tears. 'I am sorry.'

'This is just for now, Dad,' I said. 'It is just until we can sort things out for you.' I meant it then.

He cried on his single bed, in a square room with white walls, bare except for a picture of Jesus on the cross that perhaps the last patient's family had pinned up. In an effort to make myself feel better, I upgraded his room, and he was moved to one with more light, an ensuite and a TV. It took a few weeks for me to notice that he could no longer operate a remote control, nor could he understand how the TV worked. He had used a TV and a remote all his life.

Some months later, I received a call to say that he had woken up in the middle of the night, forgotten where the toilet was and peed in the middle of his room. 'He is obviously disoriented.' I fobbed the nurse off. 'I know adult men in their twenties who pee in the middle of the room when they are drunk. Just give him some time. He is not familiar with his new surroundings.'

Then, the following month, I noticed that he was wearing adult nappies. 'Why is my dad in nappies?' I enquired of the nursing staff. Their dispensing area was just across from my dad's room, so I was sure to find them organising their medicine trolley in the brown corridor on a Sunday afternoon.

'He forgets how to use the toilet sometimes,' his nurse replied politely.

I could not argue with that.

Another two months later, I was operating when I received a phone call. The circulating nurse called out the number to me, and I recognised it as the nurse manager of Dad's residential facility. 'Yes, please, can you answer it?' I asked the circulating nurse. 'Hello?' I said loudly over the din, as she held the phone to my ear.

'Hi, Ineke?'

'Yes,' I said abruptly. 'I am operating. Is there a problem?'

'Yes,' she confirmed. 'The nurses this morning went into your father's room to change him, and he had taken his nappy off and wiped his faeces all over his bedroom walls.'

Fuck. Of course, he had not done this consciously. He had simply not known what to do with his soiled nappy. Still, I was tired. 'Why are you calling me to tell me this?' I asked her, a little too aggressively.

'I just wanted to let you know,' she replied. 'Sometimes he is not co-operative with the nurses, and we have asked the doctor to see him and maybe prescribe something to calm him down.'

Correctly or not, I interpreted the nurse's voice at the other end of the phone as judgmental, and I felt like a cat ready to attack. Then I remembered the little old lady with dementia who had massaged faeces into the walls of cubicle B5 in the emergency department, and I felt acutely embarrassed about the way I had judged her. 'Thanks for calling me,' I managed to spit out.

After thanking the circulating nurse for answering and holding the phone for me, I took a deep breath, then lost myself once more in the familiar movements of operating.

* * *

As all this drama was unfolding in the dementia unit of the rest home 800 kilometres away from my theatre, I had a patient five floors up with dementia who was sitting in his hospital bed with a tube in his nose, a bag of nutrition running through his veins and an incision the length of his abdomen.

He had presented as critically unwell in the middle of the night. The nurse at his rest home had noticed him groaning in pain, and there was vomit on his dressing gown. For people such as this man, who are unable to communicate, the pathology can have been brewing for hours or days longer than it might with someone who is able to say something is wrong from the outset. We determined that his gut had perforated, meaning he must have been in terrible agony. He required an emergency operation and resection of the offending gut, but we also had to engage the intensive-care specialists because of the possibility he would require post-operative support in the ICU. This man was only 65, and had been a busy and successful engineer until he was diagnosed with early-onset Alzheimer's disease a few years earlier. He could no longer communicate, nor could he walk, but he had a family who loved him and, although they were no longer able to care for him at home, they tried as much as possible to keep him as an integral part of the family.

Although dementia should not be a discriminating factor for access to treatment, there is a large amount of discussion in the literature over the compatibility of ICU with dementia, and in particular advanced dementia. It is a logical question. When you have a patient in front of you who has no idea what is happening – who is completely ignorant of what lies ahead, who does not understand the commitment required to recover after major surgery, who might not understand pain – should you subject them to major abdominal surgery with its inherent complications, perhaps a stoma, the possibility of a return to theatre, further deconditioning, and the risk of deterioration of their already fragile neurocognition? Or is that cruel?

The American Geriatric Society does not recommend tube-feeding for patients with dementia who are no longer able to eat. The reasons for this are multiple. For one, the use of a feeding tube increases the risk of agitation, which requires restraints, chemical or physical. Then there's the risk of complications associated with a patient aspirating the feed into their lungs and causing life-threatening pneumonia and pressure ulceration.

The diagnosis of dementia brings with it a life expectancy of about three to twelve years, with some researchers reporting an increased risk of complications after surgery and thus a higher risk of early mortality. However, the presence of dementia should not be prohibitive on its own. The other factors to take into account are the existence of other medical problems, the patient's age, what they might have wanted, and finally what their family wants and thinks they might have wanted.

All these considerations are challenging to weigh up for someone who requires a life-saving operation in the middle of the night. Sometimes, people have written an advance care directive – a signed statement setting out in advance the treatment they want or do not want in the event of becoming unwell and unable to make a decision in the future – and that makes things a little easier for us, but as is usually the case there was no such guidance in this instance.

We decided very easily that, at the age of 65, with no other medical problems whatsoever, he should go under the knife. Surgery was straightforward. His colon had perforated because of a large build-up of stools in the left part of it. Sometimes when this happens, the pressure of the stools against the wall of the colon can cause what we call a stercoral perforation. It necessitated a stoma, something the nurses were going to have to manage for this man for the rest of his life, because he would never be able to understand it.

His recovery over the next few days in the ICU was straightforward. He was placed on an infusion of morphine to help control his pain, but this left him even less able to communicate than normal. And, unfortunately, from that moment on things were not so routine. On our ward round on day four after his operation, we found his bed surrounded by the resuscitation team because he was in respiratory distress. He had vomited in the middle of the night, while lying down; then, unable to communicate because of a combination of his dementia and his pain medication, he had aspirated the vomit into his lungs. This is called an aspiration pneumonia, and because of the incredibly corrosive nature of the stomach contents it has the potential to be life-threatening. He was transferred back to ICU for assistance with his breathing, and fortunately he settled without needing to be put back onto the ventilator.

A clammy-looking man ascended the elevator plastered against his bed two days later. He had been deemed well enough to exit ICU, although we were not convinced. His recovery was incredibly slow, which was no surprise. He'd had three major traumas in less than a week: a life-threatening intra-abdominal event, a major operation with a long anaesthetic, and then an aspiration pneumonia. All with a background of chronic illness. His gut stopped working with what we call a paralytic ileus, and he required nutrition through his veins and lots of time. A paralytic ileus can occur after major abdominal surgery or major illness, and means the normal electrical activity of the gut stops. This manifests as nausea, vomiting, bloating, distension, and lack of flatus and bowel motions. It can take days or weeks to recover.

Eight days later, when his gut finally started contracting again and his stoma was working, we collectively breathed a sigh of relief. For extra safety, the staff continued to nurse him bolt upright, a position we found him in every morning, with a napkin streaked with porridge over the front of his hospital gown. It looked as if the napkin had eaten more of the breakfast than he had. His nurse aide, who was supposed to be watching him, was often found reading her magazine a couple of metres from his bed.

After three weeks in hospital, very much a victim to our knives and his inability to communicate, he was discharged back to his hospital-level care residence. Victory. Or so we thought. A month later, as we were reconciling our major morbidities, a red alert sat adjacent to his name on the hospital computer system. *Deceased.* The red letters are easy to recognise, and it filled me with sadness. Had we completely violated this man in these last weeks of his life, thinking we were helping him?

* * *

A 92-year-old man came into hospital reporting severe back pain. He was on warfarin, a medication used to thin the blood. Warfarin is also known as Coumadin, and was first commercialised as a rat poison in 1948, before it was approved for medical use a few years later. It now sits on the World Health Organization's essential medications list.

There are a few reasons for a 92-year-old man to be on warfarin. It is used to treat blood clots in deep veins, or to prevent blood clots from forming in high-risk conditions. One of these conditions is when the heart is in atrial fibrillation, when the heart beats rapidly and irregularly, leading to pools of static blood in the heart. Wherever there is static blood, there is a risk of blood clotting as it pools, concentrating red blood cells and clotting factors in one place. In atrial fibrillation, the static pools of blood around the heart valves can result in the formation of clots. These clots can then embolise or be sent into the circulation, most importantly the cerebral circulation, which results in a stroke. A CHADS2 score estimates the risk of a stroke in atrial fibrillation, taking into account age, other medical problems and the history of previous stroke. This man's CHADS2 score had been sufficiently high that it was felt he should be given warfarin.

The corollary of being on a blood-thinning medication is that one bleeds easily, and a simple fall – particularly in an elderly person who is living at home alone – can be fatal if they lose their balance and knock their head. But it was back pain that this man had come in with, and as a general surgeon I was worried about a major bleed into his retroperitoneum (the area in the back of the abdomen, behind the peritoneum).

Apart from that, and in every other way, he looked wonderful. His heart rate and blood pressure were perfect. He was not sweaty. His hands were warm and his pulse full. He was thin, with no evidence of a major vessel rupture on my examination of his abdomen. He was alert and very pleasant. It was all a little strange. His X-rays were normal. There was no blood in his urine, which you might expect with a kidney stone, which can also cause severe back pain. His blood tests were normal, his blood count better than mine and his level of warfarin in the blood absolutely where it should have been. So I requested a CT scan of his abdomen, even though everything else seemed benign. He was 92 –

I had to investigate further. No surprises, his CT scan was absolutely normal. It was a mystery.

But you do not discharge a 92-year-old man who has required hospitalisation without extensive assessment of his living situation. It was a Thursday night, and the weekend was around the corner. He did not have any family, and I did not want to send him home alone over the weekend, when our social workers would not have time to assess him for home help. So I told him I would keep him in hospital for the weekend, and that I wanted a complete appraisal of his living situation to make sure he would be safe going home. He was limber and in extraordinary form for a man in his nineties, and listened politely to my explanations and engaged pleasantly. He was obviously sharp. It was an absolute pleasure for me to have him occupying a hospital bed.

Monday came, and the social worker, occupational therapist and physiotherapist saw him. He really was in great shape, and I knew this was all just an exercise, but I hated the idea of sending him home alone, even if there was no reason for him to be in hospital. We did, however, need to get him home before he caught a diarrhoea-inducing bug from the surgical ward. Moreover, beds in the hospital are always in high demand, with patients being kept in the corridors of the emergency department until beds become available when others are discharged from the ward. His paperwork was completed, and a neighbour came to pick him up and take him home.

A week later, I received a letter from the hospital. It came in one of those horrible-looking official, thick A4 envelopes we get if something bad has happened. They are usually thick because they contain a patient file. It was the hospital lawyer, asking me to detail the elderly man's admission, including the objective assessment at the time of his presentation, any investigations and any treatment in hospital. He had been found dead at home by a member of the home help team who had gone in to clean his house.

I was devastated. I had been afraid to send him home, and I regretted doing so immediately, although I'd had no good reason to keep him in hospital. Of course, at 92, living alone is a rarity, and from a humanistic point of view it seems lonely and cruel. I reviewed his notes with a fine-tooth comb, underlining all the assessments by the nurses and multidisciplinary team. I sought reassurance from a good friend and colleague who told me that the only thing I had done wrong was to request a CT scan when there had been no indication that one was necessary. Nonetheless, his death stayed with me, and I wondered what I could have done differently.

When I finally received his cause of death, I was still unsure. He had been found in his bed by a perfect stranger with a plastic bag over his head. Cause of death: suicide. Scratch that: loneliness.

* * *

Mrs A was admitted during my night on call. She was 88 years old, and the night registrar said that she was a shared admission between medicine, psychiatry and surgery — and duly bore the brunt of our displeasure for allowing such a thing to happen. The morning team is never enthused by an admission shared this way, as it often means there is no surgical problem. Nevertheless, these admissions happen more and more as we are faced with an increasingly elderly population consuming healthcare. Not only are health problems more frequent with increasing age, but polypharmacy (the prescription and use of multiple medications) comes with drug-induced complications that result in hospital admission. And, of course, there is an element of acopia — that is, elderly people who are living alone, with little to no support network, and not coping in their current living situation.

This woman had tried to commit suicide. She had taken a drug overdose, and was deemed to be medically stable, but she complained of severe abdominal pain, and the medical team was unsure what this meant in the context of her overdose. Due to her intention to commit suicide, she was also admitted under the acute psychiatric team, and had a watch by her bedside.

When I walked in, I found a despairing elderly woman lying on her side, curled in the foetal position. She was distraught. I sat by her, so that I might be able to see her face. She was in tears and, quite simply, did not want to live. She lived alone, with no family and no friends, and she was miserable and horribly lonely. She begged to be left to die. In fact, she asked for more than that – she asked us to help her die. I understood her distress, but I could not do as she wished. So I told her I understood, and that I would do everything I could to help her, then I asked for the psychiatric opinion and their assessment of her mental state. As it was, she had severe abdominal pain for which we could find no reason, and there was no doubt she was hoping that it would be a life-threatening event. After a comprehensive psychiatric assessment, we decided we would not investigate the nature of her severe abdominal pain because, whatever the outcome, she was not a good surgical candidate and it was unlikely she would survive any major abdominal surgery.

So, she was placed on a morphine syringe driver under the guidance of our palliative care service, and she died within 24 hours – probably with a sigh of relief.

* * *

I was woken at 2 a.m. – it is *always* 2 a.m. – by the night registrar to review Mrs T, a 60-year-old woman with free air on her chest X-ray, evidence that there was a perforation in the bowel. This requires surgery most of the time, but in a minority of cases we can allow time and antibiotics to heal the perforation instead. We call this conservative or non-operative management, and to be suitable for this a patient has to be well despite the presence of a perforation.

This woman was only 60 years old, but she had metastatic thyroid cancer, which had spread to her brain and lungs. She had been having radiotherapy for the brain metastases, and was on steroids to reduce swelling. In view of everything she was undergoing and the fact that she was on steroids, the air had most likely come from a stomach or a duodenal ulcer. She was unwell with systemic compromise – a rapid heart rate and low blood pressure. The registrar told me over the phone that he had already spoken to the family about palliation, as he had decided she would be best managed in this way given the context.

I, however, was not convinced that palliating her was the right thing to do. I told the registrar to call the woman's oncologist and ask about her life expectancy, and learnt it was at least six months. Six months was more time on this earth than an imminent death, which would be the case if we did nothing. 'Book her for theatre to repair a perforated ulcer,' I told the surprised registrar. 'I want her taken in immediately.'

The family, too, was taken aback. After the registrar had spoken to them, her daughter had organised an international flight for a final goodbye. I explained why we should operate, and that it had not occurred to me that they would want anything else. They agreed. Of course, if she could live for six more months that would be better than 24 hours.

Steadfast in my decision, I operated on her in the middle of the night. Fortunately, she was thin, so we could make a smaller incision, which would make a difference to her post-operative recovery – she'd have less pain, a lower risk of respiratory compromise and a quicker path to mobility. Sometimes we pat ourselves on the back for considering these small details. I washed out her abdominal cavity, sutured a patch over the hole, placed a drain adjacent to the repair just in case it leaked, and closed her up neatly. The operation was straightforward. I saw her in recovery, and told her everything had gone well, but she was still sleepy after her midnight escapades. I saw her one more time later that day, before I was off for the weekend after a week of acute call.

By Monday morning I was well recovered, feeling bright, and I began the ward round on my patients from the previous week. Alas, I could not find the woman on my list of inpatients. I went around the ward, asking the staff where she had gone, and that was when I learnt that she had died the night before. She had become acutely unwell on Sunday morning, and after a short period of aggressive resuscitation, with intravenous fluids and high-dose antibiotics, she pleaded for her treatment to stop. She could not take it anymore. She was tired, and she wanted to die. The registrar on call had spent time speaking both with her and with her family to ensure that they understood this event meant death. They understood, and it was what they wanted too. The registrar requested a palliative service review.

They moved her to a single room so she could be surrounded in quiet by her husband and children, before receiving a palliative infusion of fentanyl and midazolam – a concoction to alleviate pain, and provide mild sedation. She died peacefully in the middle of the night.

The patient and her family had been happy to choose a non-operative pathway, so why had I decided to operate on her at 2 a.m. the previous week? Was it ego? Had I made the right decision? Should I not have fought for her to have a few more months with her family? Did I persuade her and her family to have surgery against their wishes? Should I have left her in peace? So many unanswered questions.

Making a decision for acute surgery in the middle of the night, especially when there are so many factors to consider, is incredibly difficult. Even among surgeons, there are differences in opinion. What one might see as futile, another sees as worth the risk. The limits of what we can achieve and how much further we can push sometimes do not correlate with a patient's psychological and physical limits. I just hoped that I had not made my patient's last days horribly worse, and that she had been comfortable in her last moments.

* * *

Every few months, I was required to reassess my own father's resuscitation status in his hospital-level care. As he was a man in his early sixties, I was adamant that the answer should be yes. In fact, I was offended that the home should ask this question as if there was any other option.

But his condition continued to deteriorate rapidly. We never saw it coming. By the end of his first year, he could no longer independently use his private bathroom and toilet. He required assistance with all activities, including feeding. The home had no other option but to move him closer to nursing care, so he was shifted out of his 'elite' room, with its TV and ensuite, to the hospital-level part of the dementia unit. We had dreamt of taking him back to Samoa, his home, where he would be happier – but whether or not that would have been true is debatable, because it probably did not take him long to become immune to the ten or so residents who were wheeled out in their armchairs every day and left in the TV room, against the wall, vegetative.

What is certain now is that he cannot go back. Covid happened, and after two years of little interaction and no physiotherapy my father is no longer able to communicate, no longer able to walk and no longer able to feed himself. He is fully dependent, in a high-level dementia unit, in his mid-sixties. He is that same man who I saw several years ago, lying flat on his back with the TV blaring a Coca-Cola commercial, the only difference being that in my dad's room it's a CD blasting Elvis Presley. My father is the man hoisted into an armchair to be part of the TV-room spectatorship. I am glad he has no idea where he is.

One day after leaving his residence, I was having brunch with a friend underneath a sunny sky. I felt like I was living two different lives. An hour before, I had been feeding my father stewed apples in his bed; the next, I was sipping coffee in a busy waterfront café.

'So you still see your dad?' my friend asked.

'Yes, I go as often as I can. Maybe once a month.'

'What? But he was such an asshole!' she exclaimed.

'He is not the man he was,' I told her honestly. 'There is no point in being angry with him. That man is gone.'

And he was.

My friends thought that, given my relationship with him, I might feel that he did not deserve kindness and compassion. Thankfully, I never had to make a conscious decision about whether or not to care. When my father was diagnosed with dementia, he was no longer the mean man we had feared as children; he was a lost child, uncertain and apologetic. My own anger is gone, replaced with despair to see my father, who no matter his faults does not deserve to be living as he is now.

There was never any question about our responsibility to our father, although we offered it a little less freely than with our mother. Our father had been difficult, and had been loving with neither his children nor his wife. But he was a product of his own upbringing, and I do believe that he did the best that he could. Sometimes, we can only do that. It takes someone extraordinary to do better.

* * *

Several months into his admission in the dementia unit, I got a call to say that my father had been complaining of abdominal pain and had lost weight. These complaints get a general surgeon fired up, and I spent some time weighing up whether it was appropriate to investigate him. I was mindful of not letting my decision for further investigation be coloured by how our relationship had been, and how horrible I found our situation. I called a close friend. 'What do you think? Is it cruel to have him investigated?' I asked.

'I think you have to investigate him,' he replied without hesitation. 'I do not think it is our place to say otherwise. Give him to the doctor in the unit, and have him investigated.'

Fortunately, it turned out to be nothing. But now, several years down the line, with no other medical condition that will take his life sooner, I believe an acute life-threatening illness would be kind, while the idea of lifesaving treatment that involves surgery and a lengthy hospital admission is cruel.

Now, when the home asks me to fill out my father's resuscitation form, I have no doubt. I tick no. No resuscitation.

* * *

It still moves me to tears when I recall the first time that a patient asked me to stop treatment. He had been ravaged by complications resulting from the treatment for his colon cancer – surgery, chemotherapy, more surgery for metastatic disease – and had ended up malnourished and officially institutionalised because of the demands of his disease.

There was no evidence of any cancer left in his body, but he had developed surgical complications from his most recent procedure, and he was bouncing between episodes of sepsis and severe sepsis. His recovery ahead was long, and the pleasures of life had left him years ago. Multiple surgeries, endless months of chemotherapy, pump-feeding directly into his stomach for nutrition, special daily dressings for complicated wounds and complete deconditioning meant that he could no longer work. He spent more time in hospital than out of it, and he could no longer share the intimacies with his family that many men take for granted. In light of this, the fact that he was clear of cancer was of little to no consolation.

One morning on our round, he cried out in anguish and asked us to stop. He was tired. He said it quietly, shuddering through his own tears.

My throat and my heart hurt, but my head understood.

Every morning for countless weeks, at the end of our ward round we had tried to reassure him that there was no longer any trace of cancer in his body. Presumably, this should have made him happy. But there are fates worse than death. I had imagined the woman with thyroid cancer and a perforated ulcer would have relished another six months of life, but she had also had enough. So too had the gentleman with advanced dementia who had once been a high-functioning engineer.

Sometimes, the disease holds the ace of hearts.

Mr K was 50 years old, and at this incredibly young age was already bedbound. Diabetes had wreaked havoc with the nerves in his feet, and he could no longer walk. He lived at home with his son, who apparently cared for him, cooked his meals, washed him and carried him around the house. This was no easy feat, because Mr K weighed over 100 kilograms. He was a big man.

He had been admitted under my care with a severe soft-tissue infection around his anus, for which diabetes is a risk factor. In addition to having poor-quality tissue, a person with diabetes cannot fight infection as well as others because the cells of the immune system do not work as efficiently. This makes them vulnerable to infection, and means that once they develop an infection they have an increased susceptibility to becoming critically unwell. Such was the case for Mr K, who required three emergency trips to the operating room to debride the rotten tissue over his buttocks, along with high-dose, industrial-strength antibiotics to fight the bacterial infection.

We watched him closely for a couple of weeks, after which he stabilised surgically, giving us the opportunity to look at his social situation to see how we could improve it. He and his son had obviously just been coping at home. Often these events happen when a person has been teetering on the edge for a while. However, at a moment in time when diabetes can be well controlled in order to prevent its complications, no one should be bedbound at the age of 50 as a result of those complications. Neither should their child be carrying them around the house, cleaning them and cooking their meals, especially not when that child should be in the prime of their life. There was no doubt Mr K had to be able to access home help and any other service we could provide so as to improve both his quality of life and his son's.

My registrar and I were completing an afternoon ward round, tying up the events from the day, when we went to check on Mr K's wound. A young man in dark sunglasses sat by the window. It was sunny outside, and Mr K had a prime room – a cubicle with a view, and good afternoon sun that streamed directly onto his bed and, clearly, onto any visitor. The sunglasses were thus deemed acceptable.

'Can I please ask you to pop out of the room for a moment so that I can do a quick examination?' I asked the young man.

He stood up slowly, then extended his white cane before him and tapped his way out, carefully manoeuvring through the four-bed ward so as not to walk into a hospital trolley, his cane mapping out a safe path in front of him. It was not a penny dropping; it was a tonne of bricks.

'Who was that?' I asked. My question was redundant. I knew the answer.

'That's my boy,' Mr K replied proudly.

'This is your son who lives with you and carries you everywhere?' I asked, totally floored, my voice an octave higher than usual. 'He's blind?' I added in alarm, as if Mr K didn't already know.

'Yes, but my boy is strong, and sometimes I just drag myself around the house.'

Horror and disbelief are good words to describe the exchange of glances between me and the registrar.

My heart broke. We'd had the privilege of a window into this man's life. I tried to imagine why someone would not ask for help when we live in a country where he was very much entitled to it. But before I could ask the question, my registrar, who must have been wondering the same thing, answered me. Their biggest problem was paying bills. He was right. They were just trying to live. Their day-to-day worry was food, rent, electricity, and Mr K's disappearing mobility had too high an opportunity cost to invest.

We organised for Mr K to have a multitude of social assessments to see what financial and home help he could get access to, but it all seemed a small drop compared to the complexity of his life, which we would never understand.

12.

Fortune favours the bold

It had been a tough week. As well as being my call week, it was the middle of winter and the skies had let us know it. I was running late for work, and the rain was torrential. I almost couldn't see the road ahead, but the downhill route to the hospital was a familiar one. One I was very used to racing down on the way to work. Whenever I was late, I sped along that road automatically. Then a man struggling with the poor visibility as much as I was jumped out from one of the parked cars, right into the middle of the road. I screeched to a stop. His hands struck my car's bonnet as if he could have fended me off. My heart was racing. I had almost hit him. It was a sign, I told myself. A sign that I needed to slow down. Literally and figuratively.

It was Friday, the day when we try to clear as much of the emergency operative caseload as we possibly can. Some Fridays, I have been summoned to theatre because there are 50 hours of operating on the emergency board. This is in addition to the tsunami of elective operating cases across all other specialties. How, we are asked, do we plan to get through the work? It is a question that leaves me dumbfounded. Keep going, maybe?

Theatre control is always buzzing. You can have the acute co-ordinator, the head nurse co-ordinator, the duty anaesthetist and the head anaesthetic tech along with all the on-call surgeons – from general surgery, orthopaedics, neurosurgery, vascular surgery and urology – standing in front of the digital whiteboard, fighting to get their case into theatre next. Some are already in theatre attire, while others are in their suits between ward rounds and clinics. General surgery often has the biggest caseload, and on that particular day I had enough senior and junior registrars to open three theatres to clear patients who had been waiting for the better part of the week.

One of these patients was Mrs B, who was in her eighties and had presented a few days earlier with an infection in her gallbladder, which had not settled with intravenous antibiotics. She had a persistent fever, and her blood tests showed worsening infection, so we decided to push on and perform a laparoscopic cholecystectomy (keyhole removal of the gallbladder). By the time she had gone to sleep, there were already two other general surgery emergencies asleep in adjacent theatres, and I had capable registrars operating in each one.

Mrs B was tough from the outset. Her gallbladder was frozen, and it was difficult to delineate the anatomy clearly.

Several times during the operation, we wondered whether we should convert her to an open operation, but the ramifications for a woman over 80 recovering from such a big wound under her ribcage seemed excessive, and we were progressing, albeit slowly.

A call for help from the second emergency theatre added stress to an already tense situation. I scrubbed out of Mrs B's case and ran down the corridor. Fortunately, it turned out the call for help was not a major deal, and required only a pair of experienced eyes. I returned to Mrs B's theatre, rescrubbed and refocused, breathing a little faster because I felt stretched. I was picking away with my laparoscopic instruments when all of a sudden something gave way and the anatomy seemed to be clearer. It almost seemed too good to be true. We completed the operation, and I breathed a sigh of relief.

Mrs B looked well on the day immediately following surgery, and we decided to keep her in for an extra night. She was recovering from both a severe infection of her gallbladder and a long operation, so it would have been cruel to send her out so quickly. On the second day, something was amiss. We walked into Mrs B's cubicle to find that she was yellow – a horrible sight for a surgeon after a difficult gallbladder operation, and a huge problem.

For all patients undergoing any type of surgery, we go through something called informed consent, which requires a two-way dialogue between the treating doctor and the patient. The surgeon – or any treating doctor, for that matter –

is required to explain all the options for treatment (including *no* treatment), and the inherent risks and benefits, in such a manner that the patient can assimilate this information, ask questions and make an informed decision about their own healthcare. In New Zealand, a patient's code of rights ensures that this is granted to all consumers of healthcare. Informed consent came into effect after an inquiry in the late 1980s when a gynaecologist was discovered to have been performing cervical smears on women in National Women's Hospital, then failing to treat women standardly in order to observe the natural history of cervical cancer.

When we obtain consent, we discuss the most significant complications of the operation. With a laparoscopic cholecystectomy, there is a risk in one patient out of approximately 300 of inadvertent injury to the common bile duct – the tube that extends from the gallbladder to the small bowel. If the bile duct is damaged, it can have huge consequences. Repairing it requires a complex open operation through a wound under the ribcage that extends from one side of the abdomen to the other. There is also an increased risk of death, a reduced life expectancy, a long hospital stay, and multiple procedures and readmissions over the course of the patient's remaining lifetime.

I was devastated to see Mrs B jaundiced. At that point, I had performed over 800 laparoscopic cholecystectomies, and to my knowledge had never had a bile duct injury. But I sat down on the bed next to her, and explained that there had almost certainly been a complication, and I was worried that we had tied off her bile duct. Open disclosure is an important part of a surgeon's practice. It ensures that adverse consequences are disclosed to patients whenever unintended harm occurs. As I told her what the problem was, the next investigations that she would require, and the surgery ahead of her, I took stock of the surroundings, including a walking frame by Mrs B's bedside that I had not noticed before. Everything we do is associated with risk, and we know that, but, confronted with Mrs B's shade of yellow and mentally mapping her road ahead, I felt sick. She was not the fittest 80-year-old. I hoped that she would make it through the journey of her life, but I was scared that she would not.

She was transferred to the care of a specialist biliary reconstructive surgeon. Major complications like this are discussed among peers in what is called a morbidity and mortality meeting every Friday morning. The forum invites criticism and questioning, with the goal being to improve our own practice and thus improve patient outcomes. Just about every Friday for six months, we spoke about Mrs B as she underwent a series of procedures before reconstruction of her biliary tree could even be attempted, and for many of those Fridays we all thought she would not make it. I hated those Fridays.

Sometimes, we have patients who have complications with *everything*. Mrs B fell into such a group. She consistently fell into the 5 per cent minority of events not going according

245

to plan. Between surgical night-shift and morning-shift handovers, Mrs B was often reported as being in dire straits, having bled the night before or been transferred to intensive care for help with her breathing. It was an endless affair. But, miraculously, after several incredibly rocky months, the storm finally settled, and she was deemed well enough to have her bile-duct reconstruction.

Sometimes there is a very fine line between doing good and causing harm. 'There but for the grace of God go I,' a consultant said to me once when I was a very junior doctor. I did not know what it meant then, but I very much understand it now. Everything we do as surgeons is associated with risk. Although the vast majority of the time things go well, when a patient falls into the less-than-1-per-cent, we can start down a path of no return as they fight to get back to the same level of function with which they first came to hospital. Very infrequently, they might not make it out of hospital at all.

But Mrs B made it. Every day for six months, I arrived on the ward and checked to make sure she was still alive, terrified I wouldn't see her name on the whiteboard. And, six months later, when her bile duct was finally reconstructed, she put on her sneakers and walked out of hospital – without her frame.

I often think about that morning when I slammed on the brakes, stopping inches from a man walking through the rain. I could have hit him with my car. Maybe he really was a sign that I should have slowed down that day. I should have paid more attention. I should have taken stock.

* * *

I had wondered when I would stop surgery. I knew that it would have to come to an end. For all the good things that I had done and all the people I had helped, it was the stories of near misses, the complaints, the complications and the deaths that stuck. They kept me up at night. When the coroner's report for the two teenage boys who had died on the operating table, one after the other, came back saying that their injuries had been immediately fatal and non-salvageable, I was relieved that I was not responsible.

Not long after that, I found myself waiting for another coroner's report – this time, the young man with the splenic injury who was found dead in his hospital bed one morning – to help me sleep again.

I felt that I was living from one emergency to the next, but I was longing to experience my own life and my own thoughts and to share them with the people I loved. My son was in boarding school, and we treasured our weekends together, but he knew I was exhausted and he never asked for much.

My departure from surgery was coming. I knew it. I was just waiting for the moment. I was waiting for that coroner's report that would tell me I had been responsible. I loved general surgery, but I felt like I was waiting to fall on the other side of fortune.

* * *

The emergency department called to say that they had a young man with rectal prolapse and they couldn't push it back up. He was, I was informed, fit and healthy, did not live in an institution, was there with his wife and did not take any regular medication.

As I went to assess him, I mumbled to my resident that it must be haemorrhoids. Rectal prolapse is rare in a fit young man. It is more commonly seen in elderly ladies, and if it is seen in young people they generally have a background of institutionalisation. But not everyone falls into these categories. We learn in medicine that the exception to the rule is not exceptional.

In the emergency-department corridor, lying on his side on a trolley, stricken by pain, I found a huge and incredibly muscular builder. He was pale, hyperventilating and had his legs drawn up to his chest. Unfortunately, the corridor where he was lying was packed, which was only adding to his distress. I wheeled him into a vacant examination room to inspect his nether regions, and as I suspected his problem was prolapsing haemorrhoids, which can bring even the most robust of men to their knees. The man's wife sat next to him, alarmed at the degree of his discomfort, not trusting that it could be something so simple. Surely, such a small problem could not have rendered her hero so powerless.

It's the sort of spot question you might get in a consultancy exam: is this a rectal prolapse or haemorrhoids? I had once been asked the same question in a practice quiz. And I was not surprised my emergency department colleagues had thought this man's entire rectum was prolapsing. For, not only did this Goliath-like builder have prolapsing haemorrhoids that would not go back on their own, but the haemorrhoids themselves were Goliath-sized – the biggest I had ever seen. Photo-worthy. I called our photographer so that we could keep some high-quality photographs on a teaching file, and I think I still have those photos in the presentation I give to young surgical registrars.

He needed morphine, an ice pack and a helping hand – literally. 'Stay on your side and breathe in and out,' I told him as I pushed the haemorrhoids back up firmly against a tight anal sphincter, obviously hypertonic because of the local events. I felt a little David-esque with my finger in his anus, which at that moment afforded him some relief. He and his wife looked stunned as I told them we would keep him overnight to make sure he remained comfortable. 'Operating on big, engorged haemorrhoids is unpleasant and, additionally, we risk taking too much tissue with the swelling and ending up with narrowing of the anal canal,' I explained. 'So let's see if we can settle them down now, and manage this definitively later down the track.'

'Thanks so much, doc. Sorry you had to see that,' he said as I left the room.

It's my job, Goliath, I thought. Patients always apologise that we have to examine their anal canals and rectums.

Unfortunately, the next morning the man was in excruciating pain again. The haemorrhoids had dropped out when he got up to pee. We decided to operate, and several hours later, after a general anaesthetic and an open haemorrhoidectomy, he was back on the ward. When I found him and his wife in the lounge, he was much more comfortable. 'You can go home,' I told him.

He broke into a huge smile. 'Can I give you a hug, doc?' he asked.

'Only if you call me David,' I replied.

Goliath was back on his feet, albeit in a blood-stained gown, still with his faithful wife by his side.

* * *

Several years prior to her arrival at my clinic, a woman in her thirties had undergone a simple mastectomy for breast cancer with a plan to have a delayed reconstruction once treatment was complete. In lay terms, she'd had her breast removed and was left with a flat chest wall on one side.

As is often the case, once her other treatments – namely chemotherapy and radiotherapy – were complete, she had decided she wanted to get back to normal life before embarking on major surgery to reconstruct her breast. Life comes to somewhat of a standstill when you have to get through the daily demands of chemotherapy and radiotherapy, which can all last the better part of a year. For anyone, this is a long time, and it comes at a significant cost to life outside the hospital. A woman in her thirties, for instance, is forced to put things like embarking on important career opportunities, and starting new relationships or a family on hold. You could say that it is the price to pay for successfully achieving a cure, but the cost can be a significant one, and we never discount that.

Four years after the initial operation, this woman had finally decided it was time to be symmetrical in a bathing suit. In my experience, most women who get to this point after having lived for several years without a breast have altered their life to accommodate the lack of symmetry. It might be that they wear a prosthesis in their bra to match the other side, or they avoid altogether activities where they feel exposed – public pools, gym changing rooms, downward dog at yoga – or they change their wardrobe completely. This adaptability is admirable, and after a few years of such progressive lifestyle changes most are convinced that they could happily live without a breast; moreover, they understand that they are not defined by their breasts. Again, this is admirable. However, I am not defined by my nose, but I would still like my nose to stay on my face.

This particular woman presented at my clinic wishing to explore her options for reconstruction. How would it be done? What would be the cost? What were the risks? What would it look like? She had been 28 years old when she'd had her mastectomy and, while she was now successful in her career, she was not in a relationship because of a lack of self-esteem, especially sexually. She said she had been like this for so long that she had not thought of more surgery until someone else suggested it.

As is standard, we had several consultations about the operation and her expectations for recovery. She was not defined by her breasts, she said. I think this must be written somewhere on a breast-cancer survivor website, because we hear it a lot. It plays a little like a broken record. She also told me she would not do it to make herself more appealing to a man. To this, I replied that she was not doing it for a man; she was doing it for herself. And, I added, this was not a simple case of vanity. She had been born with two breasts, and it is neither shameful nor vain to desire a return to this.

After several appointments, she decided it was time to move forward, and we booked a date for surgery. Three months later, I saw her in the pre-operative bay, where she signed the consent-to-surgery form, and we proceeded with surgical marking. Using a marker, I drew first the location I would take tissue from, then the new footprint on her chest wall of the breast that this tissue would fill. No matter whether a patient has been on the waitlist for one week or six months, there is always an element of anxiety at this moment in the pre-operative assessment bay. They have to trust that, while they are asleep, defenceless, we will do our best for them.

The woman's operation took three hours, and it went well. She woke in recovery, looked down at her chest, saw for the first time a mound where for years she had been flat, and burst into tears of relief. As I watched her, the back of my throat hurt with emotion. All those years of telling herself that she could live with one breast were behind her. Denial can be a powerful thing.

* * *

In the middle of the night, a woman brought her distressed mother into hospital. She was the main carer for her mother, who was elderly and bedridden. She was also the main carer for her son, who had severe autism, and for her husband, who after serious head trauma was epileptic and could no longer work. They were refugees, and the daughter interpreted for us.

The mother had developed sudden severe pain some hours ago, and it was growing progressively worse. She had been reasonably well up until that point, eating and drinking normally, albeit bedridden and dependent on her daughter for all her daily care. Her clinical examination, blood tests and a CT scan of her abdomen suggested that she had gut ischaemia, meaning that there was a lack of blood supply to her small bowel, most likely because of a small clot. The condition is often fatal unless we operate. However, given her medical history and her poor general condition, we decided that she was not a surgical candidate. This meant that we were going to allow her to succumb to this event. She was placed on a morphine pump and I explained to the daughter that the goal was to keep her mother comfortable, and that her mother would likely die within 48 hours, although it is always difficult to be exact with time. The daughter acknowledged this sorrowfully, and the family moved into a single room overnight.

On the first morning, the mother was unresponsive, but evidently comfortable, and we explained again to the daughter her likely diagnosis, and that we were at the family's disposal if she had any concerns.

On the second morning, her mother was equally unresponsive – no worse, no better – and again we expressed that our main goal was to keep the mother comfortable. It was nothing out of the ordinary. Sometimes the demise can be quick, and sometimes it can take a little longer – a couple of days, a week. We can never be absolutely sure.

On the third day, she rose again. I had gone straight to theatre in the morning instead of rounding on the ward patients, and was surprised early that afternoon when my resident asked if we should restart fluids and antibiotics for the woman we were palliating. Once we palliate someone, we usually stop antibiotics or any other interventions that might be considered active treatment. Instead, we give pain relief or sedation, but we stop their usual blood-pressure medication and whatever else they might have been on. 'Do you know what palliation means?' I asked him, giving him a look that expressed how ridiculous I thought his question was. Nervous silence. 'Why on earth would we restart antibiotics and steroids for a lady who is going to die?' I persisted when I did not get an answer.

'She became more alert overnight, and had breakfast with her family this morning,' he told me sheepishly.

We exchanged looks, and he nodded as if to reassure me that I had indeed heard correctly.

By later that afternoon, the palliative care team phoned us in theatre to say that the woman had woken up completely. Surprised, I went to the ward, and found the family rejoicing and praising the lord, Jesus Christ. The mother had opened her eyes early that morning, and had recognised each and every one of them. She had told them that she was hungry, so her daughter had gone out to get a McDonald's milkshake. A breakfast of champions.

By day four she was eating toast and an omelette for breakfast, and on day five she was being wheeled out of hospital on a trolley after we had removed her intravenous line, nasogastric tube and urinary catheter. She and her family thought it was nothing short of God's miracle.

Us? We were happy, as we always are when our patients are happy – and alive.

The further you go in surgery, the more you learn that nothing is the rule. A 20-year-old gets terminal bowel cancer, while the 90-year-old you are sure is going to die doesn't. Surgeons are only human. We get it wrong sometimes, too. And sometimes we get it really wrong. This job keeps you humble.

* * *

Mr G was transferred from a private hospital four days after a hip-joint replacement. He had severe abdominal pain and free air on a chest X-ray, which you may recall is indicative of a perforated ulcer. In Mr G's case, this was probably a result of the non-steroidal, anti-inflammatory pain relief he had no doubt been using for joint pain.

Since Mr G weighed 140 kilograms, we also took a CT scan, just to make sure the hole was, in fact, in the top half of his abdominal cavity rather than the bottom. He had a lot of fluid and inflammation around his stomach, and the CT scan allowed us to focus the incision where it had to be, rather than making a very large cut over a very large abdominal wall as if we were performing an exploratory procedure. The hole was easily found, and it was exactly where we expected it to be: over the first part of the duodenum, just beyond the stomach. There was a round, punched-out ulcer with at least two litres of green gastric content bathing his gut. Green gastric fluid should be inside the stomach, not sitting outside it. We washed Mr G's abdominal cavity with copious amounts of warm saline –

ten litres, to be exact – put several large sutures around the hole, brought up a tongue of fat from within the abdominal cavity to plug the hole, and pulled the sutures closed. We placed two large drains next to the repair so that, if the repair leaked, we would be able to see it straightaway, and also so that any leaked gastric content would drain straight out of his abdominal cavity rather than accumulating and making him seriously unwell. We were pleased with our repair, and we closed his very large abdominal wall.

Day one and two passed without incident. Every day that we walked in, we would find Mr G sitting up in bed, smiling. 'How are you?' he would ask.

'Great,' I would answer. 'And you? How are you doing?'

'Yeah, really good,' he would reply.

This was our morning ritual. Mr G always had a smile on his face and a tube in his nose. Since his drains were clean, and he was drinking water, we decided to remove one drain.

But on day three, before Mr G and I could run through our routine, one of the registrars pointed to the drain. There was over a litre of gastric content in the drain bag, suggesting a leak. The air was sucked out of me – and, I am sure, out of both registrars in the room. Mr G was breathing a little quicker, and he had a fever, suggesting that the leak was having an impact on his systemic wellness. 'We have to go back to theatre now,' I told the team.

Then I explained to Mr G that it seemed the repair had failed, and he was leaking gastric content again. 'Given the volume that is draining and the early signs of systemic upset, we would be better to address the problem immediately,' I said. He was calm and accepted this news without question.

Once he was asleep in theatre, we opened the staple line on his skin and the stitches holding the abdominal wall together underneath. As is usually the case in a return to theatre, things didn't open as well as they did the first time. The tissue was fragile, friable and broke with little manipulation. Everything was a little stuck, because the normal post-surgery inflammatory reaction – which is responsible for scar formation – was in evolution. Going back to theatre for any patient is tough, let alone a man who weighs 140 kilograms. It is always a fine balance between solving the problem and not making things worse during these returns to theatre.

Mr G had green gastric content sitting in the upper part of his abdomen, so we cleaned that out, then inspected the site carefully to see where the content had come from. We lifted the liver to inspect our repair, and surprisingly it was intact. We flipped the stomach back and forth to see if, perhaps, we had missed another ulcer. We extended the incision to make sure we were not missing a leak from elsewhere, but the bottom half of his abdomen was pristine. It was so pristine, in fact, that we risked spreading infected fluid from the top part of his abdomen to the bottom and potentially causing future problems. We filled his abdominal cavity with saline and pumped air into his stomach to see if the fluid would bubble and thereby prove that there was a leak if the air escaped. Zero. We could not find another leak anywhere.

Defeated, we placed another couple of drains, and closed him again. Then we asked the anaesthetist to place an intravenous line that would run from his neck to the top part of his heart for nutrition, because he would be strictly nil by mouth until we knew he was stable.

Had we done Mr G any favours by taking him back? I wasn't sure. Regardless, the next morning Mr G was sitting upright with a smile on his face and the tube in his nose. He also had a big bag of nutrition through his veins.

'How are you?' he asked, as I entered the room.

'Great, Mr G,' I replied. 'How are you doing?'

'Yeah, really good,' he replied.

For two more weeks, we continued to exchange this dialogue every morning, and meanwhile the drains became more clear than green. Finally, after another scan, we felt close to brave enough to remove one of the drains. We pushed blue dye through the tube in Mr G's nose to make sure it did not come out of one of the drains. Hoorah! No blue in the drains, so he could drink again.

The final hiccup was to be expected for an obese man who has undergone two abdominal operations. His abdominal wound had to be reopened because of infection, and a special dressing had to be placed to protect the wound and accelerate healing – yet another attachment, but one that would not keep Mr G in hospital.

The last time I saw him, he was lying in bed with his abdominal wound exposed and being dressed by our specialist wound nurse.

'How are you?' he asked.

'Great, Mr G. And you?'

'Yeah, really good,' he replied.

Later that day, after four weeks in hospital, Mr G walked out of hospital with one drain attached to his abdominal wall, no tube in his nose, still with the smile on his face and, of course, his new right hip. Perhaps he was also a few kilograms lighter.

* * *

I first met 90-year-old Mr P at the end of a long Saturday spent in the acute operating theatre. After developing central abdominal pain that afternoon, he had called his daughter late in the evening because the pain was escalating in severity. He had then been brought into hospital by an ambulance, accompanied by his children. Mr P was in great shape and had never seen the inside of a hospital apart from during the birth of said children. He lived alone on a farm, where he continued to actively manage the property.

When he arrived, he had all the signs of a man with an abdominal catastrophe. He was extremely distressed with pain and required large amounts of morphine, which offered very little relief. He was dehydrated, and his heart rate was rapid. His abdominal examination was unremarkable. We could not elicit any point of tenderness, but he was distressed. We describe this as 'pain out of proportion to clinical findings', and it usually denotes a blood supply problem. His blood tests suggested he had gut ischaemia (a lack of blood supply to the bowel), and the X-rays looked as if he had an obstruction.

As I've mentioned, gut ischaemia can be a life-ending event. Plus, reserves are lower in older age. No matter how fit a 90-year-old person is, it can be difficult to recover from even a small knock. This, however, was not a small knock. Mr P had suffered two large knocks: a life-threatening event, and he required major surgery. He was also fiercely independent, and his children were adamant that their father would only want to survive if he could return to the same level of independence as before. We can never guarantee this, of course, although it is always the goal. He had a small window in which we could offer treatment to achieve the best chance of this happening, but it was not clear whether we were in that window or not. The more vulnerable the patient, the shorter the window is.

We decided to put a laparoscopic camera into his abdomen to assess the extent of pathology and decide whether this event was survivable. In this way, we could perform a quick diagnostic procedure through a minimal incision, without committing Mr P to a big, but potentially futile, abdominal incision. This initial laparoscopy demonstrated a central loop of small gut that had a band of scar tissue strangling it. Initially, arterial blood can still supply this loop with blood, but then the blood cannot drain out. Eventually, the pressure of accumulating blood in the affected loop exceeds the pressure of oxygenated blood flowing into this bowel, so that it becomes congested and eventually dies. The 120-centimetre section of central gut was deep red, but not dead at that moment; it was borderline salvageable.

So, we converted Mr P to an open incision and delivered the gut. The problem required a simple division of the offending band to release the gut – this was done simply with a pair of scissors. Then we had to decide whether the gut would survive or not. We placed a warm sponge over it, and waited 15 minutes to observe any change. It improved and, although it was still slightly questionable, we decided that it would be safer to leave his gut intact and give him time to recover than to resect it and confer the risk of having a leak if the two bowel ends did not heal. But we would need to watch him incredibly closely. We closed him up just after midnight, and he was returned to the ward.

His adult children were standing around his bed the next morning, as we discussed his operative findings and his expectation for recovery. Ultimately, Mr P sailed through his recovery without a hitch. We prepared him for some time in rehabilitation, thinking that he would require a period of convalescence. However, after telling us he would not need it, he then set about proving it. After less than a week in hospital, he was walking circles around the ward, and was eating and drinking normally. His bowels had opened, and on the general surgical ward this means you can go home.

He walked out of hospital on day six, surrounded by his family, looking very much the dapper man that he had been before his illness. For him, we had snuck in that window.

Better to be lucky than good, I was once told.

* * *

Mr S was brought into the emergency department with severe abdominal pain. He was Polynesian, in his sixties, robust, with traditional tattoos extending from his knees up and over his buttocks and abdominal wall.

His bowel habit had changed over the last week: he had not passed a solid motion for days, and now was not even farting. For Mr S, the change had been relatively acute, as he had been well up until the last week. Now he was in severe, unrelenting pain and could not get comfortable.

A CT scan of his abdomen showed a blockage of the left side of his colon. He had a focal area of thickening of his left colon that looked like an apple-core constriction. It was very suggestive of a cancer. On a positive note, there was no other evidence on the scan that the cancer had spread. His liver was clear, and so was his chest. That, at least, was good news.

When I spoke to Mr S and his family, I tried to convey that, despite the malignant obstruction that was evident in his colon, the goal was cure, given that the disease was localised to this small segment of the colon. However, he needed urgent surgery, because he was completely obstructed, and if it was left too long it could lead to a perforation upstream. Mr S and his family were in tears – naturally. Being told in the emergency department of a probable cancer and the need for urgent surgery is distressing.

We consented Mr S for surgery, and I saw him again in the operating theatre just before he went off to sleep. He was a big man, over 120 kilograms, and his habitus made surgery a little difficult. However, we resected the colon, re-joined him and closed him up. He most definitely had an obstruction, but other than that we could not definitively say whether there was an underlying cancer or not. We would have to wait for the pathologist to examine the specimen under the microscope.

Once he was awake and comfortable, Mr S returned to the ward, and progressed as expected during the early days after his major abdominal surgery. By day five, however, things were not quite so reassuring. His temperature was up, his abdomen was distended and he was breathing a little faster. Our primary worry was that the two ends of bowel that had been sutured together were not healing as expected, and that there may be a leak of faecal content. His blood tests showed that his inflammatory markers had sky-rocketed. After excluding his chest, urine and wound as possible sources for the change in his condition, we ran him through the CT scanner. He had a few bubbles of air outside the colon, adjacent to the anastomosis (colonic join), and free fluid. We would have to go back to theatre. Shit.

We had another meeting with his family, who were always in attendance, prior to his return and just as the pathology results landed in our laps. No cancer. The obstruction had been caused by a short segment diverticulitis, which was completely inflammatory and, most importantly, benign. Mr S and his family erupted in tears of gratitude. It was not a cancer, and this was the most important news to them. They were not perturbed that he had to go back to theatre. They huddled in prayer to thank God for this gift. Of course, Mr S still had an important surgical problem from which he could become critically unwell – but this was a much smaller detail for them.

We took him down to theatre shortly afterwards. The leak was gas only, but he did have a large amount of inflammatory fluid, and we decided to bring out a stoma upstream so that faecal material would exit into a bag, allowing the join to heal without effluent transiting it. Mr S had a rocky course after this, and required a stay in ICU, but he improved progressively and by day nine after his second operation was finally ready to go home. On the morning of his departure, his family walked in with platters of fresh baking and the most decadent chocolates. Their eyes were wet with tears as they expressed their gratitude that the head of their family – husband, father and grandfather – did not have a bowel cancer.

I told them they were more accurate to give thanks in their prayers, because I was not responsible for this. My discomfort with such an overt demonstration of gratitude overwhelmed me, and I could not eat the cakes or the chocolates that day. I had told the family it was likely a cancer when it had not been, and under my care Mr S had required a second operation and a longer hospital stay. I felt fraudulent accepting their gratitude. It took me a few days before I was able to stomach the box of chocolates I had stashed away in the office for safekeeping.

13.

How do you say goodbye?

I was on a lunch break in the middle of an all-day clinic when I walked past a nurse who stopped me in the corridor. 'You probably don't remember me,' she began, 'but I was the hospice nurse when –'

'I know, I remember,' I interrupted, then said the name of a woman we had both cared for. It had been 12 months, but I could not forget her. She had been 36 years old when she presented in May and the on-call surgeon had taken her to theatre to resect a very large left-sided colon cancer that had already spread through the wall of the colon and into the lymph nodes. When examined under the microscope, the cancer was a very aggressive cancer, but we had already known that.

The evolution of what we can achieve with surgery and chemotherapy in colon cancer meant that her medical and surgical teams were still hopeful for a chance at cure. Her pre-surgery scan had also demonstrated a single spot of cancer in the liver, and it was deemed resectable, but she required six months of chemotherapy before that could take place, and she could not start the chemotherapy until she had recovered from the emergency operation.

This woman was married with three young children under the age of eight. She wanted to live to see her kids grow up, and her goal was to get to chemotherapy. When I met her two months later, in July, she had barely left hospital. In fact, she had not made it home at all, and had been in the hospice because of intractable pain that her doctors had struggled to get under control. She had not started chemotherapy, either. I was called to see her because she had become acutely unwell with abdominal distension and pain.

A repeat CT scan demonstrated that her liver was now packed with metastatic disease, and her abdominal cavity was also full of cancer. Furthermore, her old colonic join from two months prior was leaking. She had an obstruction in her pelvis, which is probably why the leak had happened, as the obstruction downstream would have caused a blow-out at the point of weakness – the recent anastomosis.

Her referring doctor from the emergency department had told her she needed surgery, but I was going down to tell her that there was in fact nothing we could do. This was the end of the road for her. It was a horrible situation. It is always a horrible situation. Every time. No matter who. No matter how many times you have done it. I called her oncologist to make sure that there was nothing I was missing, that chemotherapy was well and truly off the cards. I also found a more experienced surgical colleague in case there was anything he could see that might help her to get out of trouble. Perhaps there was something that I had failed to think of? Sometimes, even when we already know the answers, it's necessary to share the weight of the decision. I already knew there was nothing that we could do, but I did not want to be the only one to decide that.

She was angry with me, furious, and asked me to leave. Of course, for two months, she had been single-mindedly trying to get to chemotherapy, and then to liver surgery, which was her only chance for cure. Now, here I was, telling her there was no chance for any of that to happen. She had never met me and, after everyone had told her she was going to have chemotherapy and then surgery, I was suddenly telling her that none of that was going to happen. I was telling her that the event that had brought her into hospital was likely to be terminal. Imminently.

It is no wonder that sometimes our patients do not trust us, especially when the information that we deliver is completely at odds with what they have been told previously. I apologised feebly to her, and before I left her and her husband alone, I told them I would come back the following morning to chat more with them both.

The next morning, the hospice nurses were there too. I went over her scans and her symptoms again. I explained that surgery would not help her, that it would only make her worse and take time away from her, her husband and their children. I explained that chemotherapy was not an option because it was too late. One has to be well to get through chemotherapy. That was no longer her.

'What am I going to tell my children?' she asked. 'And how much time do I have left?'

'It is always hard to say,' I replied carefully, 'but it is measured in days, and at best two to three weeks.' My own voice cracked as I said this.

We spoke about pain, and how that could be controlled. She wanted to remain alert, so as to be present with her children. She was preoccupied with food, and what she should eat, and her bowels, and how she could keep them moving. It is very common for people to be preoccupied with this, as if it is the last anchor of control.

She died ten days later in the hospice, and I knew when it happened. I never forgot about her. I could never forget about her.

All of this I remembered when the hospice nurse stopped me in the corridor. 'You did a really good job with her,' the nurse said, as we stood outside my clinic door. Her remark surprised me, because I had never felt that way. It had been a high-stress situation at a moment when the woman should have been spending time with her husband and children.

As I reflected on her that afternoon, following my encounter with her nurse, I found myself hoping that I had been able to comfort her. I remembered her because she had been so angry, almost inconsolable, and I had hoped that she had spent her last days with her family. Time had been stolen from them since her emergency surgery two months earlier, and her anger at not being able to get to chemotherapy meant that she risked not being able to find peace in her last days.

Hers was an incredibly sad story, and it made me reflect on how, for many of our patients, our ability to be compassionate and human supersedes our ability to operate. Surgical skill can be taught; only a few surgeons are naturally talented, and the rest of us can learn how to operate. The difference that surgeons can make in the lives of those we care for therefore comes down to what we all need as humans: empathy.

* * *

In life as in work, we all aim to become better people and to minimise harm to others, but sometimes small acts of kindness can make all the difference. And, in the middle of an overwhelmingly busy ward round over eight hospital floors, to watch such kindness and humanity come from a younger doctor is humbling. Is it something we lose along the way?

We were called to a medical ward to review an elderly woman with dementia who had complained of abdominal pain. She was not an operative candidate, because of all her other medical problems, but the physicians requested a surgical review to confirm a diagnosis and to document clearly whether or not she would be a surgical patient. I must admit these are not my favourite requests for review. The medical wards are often a mess – overfilled and busy. Moreover, it can seem superfluous to have to document something that is already evident. Nonetheless, to support our colleagues, we got onto it at the end of the ward round.

This woman had terrible heart failure, and we were sure that was her main problem. Quite simply, the heart has inflow and outflow, and when there is very little blood moving out, back pressure develops and fluid can pool in the lungs, the liver and the rest of the body. When it pools in the liver, the distension of the organ itself can cause liver congestion and pain. As per usual, we thoroughly assessed her admission notes, her blood tests, and any imaging she might have had in the last 24 hours and over the last years to see if we could document evolution.

Once we had completed all our detective work, we went to see her. I had two male registrars accompanying me on the ward round that morning. The patient was a little confused, and she denied abdominal pain. Her abdomen was soft when we gently palpated it in the nine segments in which we are trained to divide it, and it was obvious there was no major surgical catastrophe in evolution there. She had tenderness over her liver, and it was enlarged, which suggested that the problem had arisen because of heart failure. A simple ultrasound would confirm this, and ensure it was not because of any other infiltrative process, such as a metastatic cancer.

She was not tender anywhere else, but she was distended. So, as part of a complete gastrointestinal-tract-system examination, we turned her on her side to perform a rectal examination. As I have already said, if you don't put your finger in it, you will put your foot in it. She was wearing an adult nappy, and it was full of stools. She desperately needed to be cleaned, so I walked out of the cubicle to find a nurse to do the job. Before I could, however, my senior registrar appeared from the sluice room, holding a basin of warm water and the appropriate towels. He got on his knees, washed her, cleaned her and changed her nappy.

I was incredibly moved by his kindness and profound humility. He was exhibiting one of the key requirements of our job: humanity. A quality that cannot be acquired, unlike knowledge and surgical skill.

* * *

One of my best friends taught me how to remove an appendix. Theatre was tense when we both held instruments over the same patient. I remember him saying, 'Don't take that tone with me.' I had been impatient and become flustered during a case that was taking far too long. Regardless, he was my best ally during training – you need allies, and we are the best of friends now. Lifelong friendships often evolve during this period of training.

Another dear friend, JT, is a surgeon. We trained at the same time, but I finished before him, and he became my senior registrar just before he sat his consultancy exams. I believe I taught him how to drain pus when he was brand new. Now he takes out colons.

If I ever encountered patients after they had met JT, they never stopped speaking wistfully about him. Sure, he has bright blue eyes, but even so I thought it was clearly a case of women appreciating male doctors more than their female counterparts. One day before our 7 a.m. surgical-handover meeting, JT scrambled into the registrars' office with seconds to spare. He looked rushed, and was carrying a cake. 'What's this for?' I asked him.

'It's Mrs K's birthday cake,' he replied.

'Who is Mrs K?' I asked.

'Our patient. It's her birthday today.'

I was dumbstruck. JT, a dear friend, colleague, son of a superstar surgeon and a product of one of the most elite private schools in New Zealand, is also one of the nicest guys I know. No wonder his patients loved him. He brought them cake for their birthday if they were in hospital. I only remembered patients' birthdays if they fell on the seventh of May (mine).

* * *

One of the most rewarding aspects of being a general and cancer surgeon is meeting people. We encounter people from all walks of life, and hence we have the opportunity to learn about others. Personally, I have met thousands of people in my time as a medical professional.

We really do see all sorts, from patients who are in for minor ailments requiring simple reassurance or perhaps 24 hours of observation, to patients who need life-saving surgery for acute catastrophic events or trauma. Every patient has their story, and this is what I love. Our patients are so brave, and they endure a lot. We accompany them at moments of pain and suffering, at all stages of their treatment – diagnosis, surgery and recovery.

Cancer treatment pathways, in particular, are long. Surgeries can be complex and multiple. The journey together can be years. In all these stories of trauma, or catastrophe, or cancer we are constantly confronted by limits: of care, of what modern medicine or surgery can provide, of what the human body can sustain, of what we as medical professionals with our own stories can give, of ability, of the human soul. And after years in the job, I believe that all this is, in fact, limitless. We continue to push, and fight, and try for better. It is a crusade that must never end, because the alternative leads to mediocrity and complacency.

I have been so fortunate to witness the endless bravery in our patients, who are at the centre of it all. I hope that, for all the patients I have had the privilege of accompanying, that I made a positive contribution to their lives.

* * *

One normal Friday, when I was sitting in our weekly departmental meeting, we were talking about the same issues that we had spoken about the week before, and the week before that. I had been in this job for several years, and we were all still complaining of the same issues. They were problems that made our job to keep patients safe more difficult, resulting in changes to standard treatment pathways. I had joked to a colleague that he should wake me if someone said something different.

Suddenly, then and there, I decided that it was time to go. I was done. I could not sit in any more meetings that made no difference. I could not stand in the shower again, wrecked, wondering when I would leave. I could not live the same day repeatedly. Two months later, I handed in my resignation.

In truth, my threshold to departure was already low. In particular, there had been two recent moments, after very difficult acute surgical days with patient deaths, when I had wondered very consciously when I might leave.

There is no doubt that we all give our lives to this profession. I remember when I was just a second-year doctor working in a liver unit and one of the senior surgeons was, devastatingly, diagnosed with a bile-duct cancer. It was a cruel irony that a liver surgeon should develop a non-curable cancer of the sort standardly managed by liver surgeons. At his funeral, his children said their lasting memory of their father was watching him race along the sidelines of their Saturday-morning sports games, trying to catch the end of the match, late because he'd been at the hospital rounding on his post-operative patients. Another colleague whose wife died in the emergency department after a trauma called his secretary to cancel his clinic and quickly go through the patients who were urgent and could not wait long.

'Do you take your work home with you?' my son's psychologist asked me once.

I felt as if I was being judged. 'Yes,' I answered honestly. 'Everything is compared to what we see every day, and sometimes I go home just grateful to be alive.' I didn't appreciate her silence after that.

Our families are long familiar with being placed second to this job, second to our patients and our patients' families. The system pressures are extraordinary. There is an expectation to do more with less – to see more patients without the clinic space or support, to operate more without extra operating lists. Patient expectation is also increasing, and within this milieu we are expected to continue to minimise clinical risk.

So, no doubt we dedicate our lives to our work, and we all start out idealistic and passionate to make a difference, but eventually fatigue replaces our enthusiasm. I knew I was tired when I started to lack compassion. That was when I knew I had to take a break. I was living in a crazy balance between sadness, anger and happiness, between my family and the job, but I knew I couldn't do it all anymore. I had to choose happiness.

* * *

It has always bothered me that I could never find quite the right words to say goodbye when I knew that I would not see a patient again. One particular day, I watched my friend and colleague round on a patient with pancreatic cancer that had recurred; the patient was deteriorating quickly, and would be moved to the inpatient hospice that afternoon. 'Sadly, our paths won't cross again,' my friend said to his patient sombrely. 'But it was my absolute pleasure to have known you.'

Funnily enough, it was a patient who said something similar to me shortly afterwards. I was the on-call general surgeon, and had been handed a patient on the haematology ward who had an acute leukemia that had been diagnosed just the week before and, unfortunately, was going to be a terminal event within a matter of days. He had been fit and healthy the week before, but had presented with a fever and unwellness. He had a severe infection, which had unmasked the haematological cancer, but because of the leukemia his body could not fight it. We could not help him, as much as we wanted to. We had been speaking about the case in our Friday meeting, and everyone commented on how horrible it was. 'It's nasty,' the duty surgeon told the meeting.

278

I visited the patient on a Saturday. I walked into his cubicle, and was stunned to find that he was the husband of a breast-cancer patient I had operated on the month before. She was waiting to get on to the next part of her own cancer treatment, but obviously it had taken a back seat because of the current events. I was shocked and saddened, and I had no words. Nor did they. I explained that we could not help him, and reiterated the prognosis that the haematologists had already outlined for them. 'I'm sorry I don't have better news,' I said. 'I'm sorry that we cannot help, and for the situation in which you find yourselves.'

He was leaving that day – going home to die – with his wife and children. It was expected to be quick. Even though I have done it many times before, it is always strange to say goodbye to a patient who I know will no longer be here in a matter of days. Before I could break the silence, he jumped in. 'Doctor,' he said. 'Thank you for looking after my wife. Our paths won't cross again, but I am grateful to have met you.'

Epilogue

Two months after my mother died, I was driving in the middle of summer. The sun was shining, and I could see people running and laughing. Things you expect people to do when the sun is shining. I watched them for a moment, wondering if I would ever feel light in the sunshine again. Nothing prepares you for losing your mother, not even a career in medicine.

Sometime near the end of my surgical career, I held the hand of a patient, as I often did, while she was being drifted off to sleep. Not uncommonly, patients cry as a result of fear and stress, and this woman had tears rolling down her cheeks as the anaesthetist put the mask over her mouth and nose. 'Think of somewhere you would rather be,' the anaesthetist said to her, and for some reason I was hit so violently by guilt over not having been a better daughter, over not having accompanied my mother better through her battle against cancer. I was relieved surgery was coming to an end for me.

As time has passed, I realise that the goodness I have in me is her, and I am grateful to have had her in my life. I look at my five siblings, of whom I am the eldest, and I know that they too are wonderful people because of her. I do not mention her sisters and brothers enough, but in fact they had such a huge influence on our lives and on my mother's happiness, and they are amazingly kind, loving people, which is because of their own mother in turn.

I am grateful to my son for being patient with me. He left science and maths early, happy to be as different from his mother as he could possibly be, and is currently a student at one of the best arts universities in the world. He is brave and gentle, and he made me better. He made my life worth something. That he still thinks the world of his own mother is a miracle. One day, I had to cancel dinner with him because I had a sick patient. 'I am so sorry,' I said, followed by the eternal promise to make up for it later. Then I asked if he was okay. He looked at me and said, 'Mum, I am not the one who is sick.' Where did my child learn such compassion? Did I teach it to him? Was it fair that he compared his own needs or expectations with those of my work? I don't believe it was fair, but I do believe that he learnt compassion from the village that raised him: my mother and my siblings taught him kindness and attention to others. He is the kid who will open a door for others and help a stranger with their shopping bags.

Now, when the sun shines, I remember what my mother said to me on her last night in our home in New Zealand:

'When the clouds part, and the sun shines through them, that will be me.' I wonder if she is up there.

Only now do I see the beauty in our family.

* * *

I started writing this book as somewhat of a catharsis. I have spent the end of many on-call periods in tears of sadness and fatigue, and I still think of the many patients I have had the privilege of meeting who are no longer on this earth. What I have always found it hard to come to terms with is human vulnerability, and how life can change in an instant − be it from trauma, a life-threatening medical event or a cancer diagnosis. Over the last ten years, as I have fought through both my own parents' illnesses and journeyed with patients through theirs, the sadness of all of these stories has dug a little deeper, until it has become a large part of what I carry.

I often sat down to write about my patients when I was sad, and that is why a lot of these stories are heavy. But it is important to understand that most stories a general surgeon sees are not sad. Most end well. With modern medicine, advances in technology, and improvements in surgical techniques and perioperative care (including ICU), most stories have happy endings. The sad stories in this book represent the minority of my patients, but of course these are the stories I carry with me.

The stories I've shared come largely from personal experience, but a few were shared with me by colleagues. For those stories, I sought permission from the original surgeon. Other stories still are a montage of many similar stories. What these stories all have in common is the fact that they're the ones that kept me awake at night, wondering if and how I could have done better. They are the stories that made me realise how lucky I was to be healthy, to have a roof over my head, to have people who love me.

* * *

At the same time that I left the public hospital where I was working, so did the only other female general surgeon. That meant that, in total, three female surgeons had left the department in 12 months. There were no other female general surgeons remaining.

While writing this book, I was quite aware that I often identified whether registrars or consultants were women or men. I did so where relevant in order to demonstrate the very masculine culture in which surgeons still practise, and how that contributes to historic perceptions among patients and staff, and allows unacceptable behaviour to persist. Female surgeons are an important and vital part of the workforce, yet the growing body of research comparing outcomes for female surgeons versus their male counterparts illustrates that male surgeons are still seen as the gold standard – regardless of what actual patient outcomes suggest.

One of the things that inspired me to write this book was the simple fact that the vast majority of surgical memoirs have been written by male surgeons, many of whom portray a godliness in the profession which might have existed at another moment but prevails no longer. Furthermore, female surgeons in particular have a reputation of being cold, for many reasons. This could not be further from the truth.

Another thing that inspired me? My patients. As surgeons, we are so privileged to be part of so many special stories. Our patients are so brave, they go through so much, and not enough is ever said about their plight.

I hope this book demonstrates the breadth of what we see as surgeons, the bravery of the patients we treat, and offers a glimpse into the heart of many a treating professional.

* * *

One day, I was in my breast clinic, counselling a patient about reconstruction, going through my usual blurb about surgery – the whys, the why-nots, the risks and the benefits – when she said to me, 'You sound exactly like Dr Krishna Clough.'

'What?' I replied, taken aback.

'You sound exactly like Dr Krishna Clough,' she repeated.

'Why are you saying that to me?' I asked pointedly.

'Have you heard of him?' she said. 'He's a French surgeon. I watched his video last night. You talk just like him. Like, copy–paste.'

I broke out laughing. 'He is my husband,' I explained to my confused-looking patient.

Krishna and I met in a meeting. He was lecturing at a breast-surgery conference, and is, I think, the only man who looks sexy in a pink shirt. Some people say he looks like Daniel Craig. After that meeting, he told me a story about princesses and cowboys, and how they should not work together. I think I was the princess, and I was hooked. He lived in Paris, and we spent a few crazy years flying across the world to one another, or meeting in the middle – Los Angeles, San Francisco, Japan, Hong Kong, Singapore.

Krishna operated 14-hour lists three times a week, and had consulting days that were even longer. When we had been together two years, I asked him how he had done it for so long. 'We have a very special job,' he said. 'If I can help someone, and if I can be useful, then I will keep doing it.'

Not long after this, we were having coffee in the sun on a typical Parisian terrace, when I told him, 'I think there is a market for dog skincare. And I think I am going to go for it.'

He looked at me incredulously. I should say that the comment was not entirely out of the blue. My own dog had skin problems, and I had been making skincare with the help of a laboratory. I had also taken on a business coach and done a lot of market research.

'I love you, my wife,' he replied, 'but I think you should finish your coffee.'

I now live in Paris. Who would have thought that a girl from the South Pacific, sleeping in a single room with her parents and three other siblings, would one day become a surgeon, then stop being a surgeon, then start a new business in the city of lights?

Acknowledgements

I loved surgery. My extraordinary time in training and time on the job is due in no small part to my registrars and colleagues. I have worked with some awesome registrars – male and female – and they are amazing surgeons: Dr Stephanie Manning, Dr Bridget Watson, Dr Yu Kai Lim, Dr Sean Seo, Dr Anantha Narayanan and Dr Will Fleischl.

In particular, for my development as a surgeon, Dr Mark Grant and Dr Siraj Rajaratnam, who were instrumental in my training, helping me to complete my first appendicectomy and hernia operation independently (huge feats for a young trainee); they always told me to have confidence in myself. Professor Elizabeth Dennett, colorectal surgeon, and a member of the truth and justice league, forceful in compassion and skill, always had my back. She told me not to be a shrinking violet. Dr Chris Thorn, anaesthetist, who probably never knew the impact he had on me, but he is extraordinary with patients, so much so that I could almost do a downward dog as I listen to him send patients off to sleep. Incidentally, he is the one who said, 'You got this,' as I was embarking on my first major case as a consultant surgeon.

Ullrich, my gentle son, who never complained when his own needs were sacrificed so that I could be a better surgeon.

And my husband, Dr Krishna B Clough, world-renowned breast-cancer surgeon, who altered my universe of thought, and with whom I share all these moments.

Bibliography

A. Arnold-Foster, '"A Small Cemetery": Death and dying in the contemporary British operating theatre', Medical Humanities, 2020, vol. 46, no. 3, pp. 278–287.

M. I. Bellini et al, 'A Woman's Place Is in Theatre: Women's perceptions and experiences of working in surgery from the Association of Surgeons of Great Britain and Ireland Women in Surgery Working Group', BMJ Open, 2019, vol. 9, no. 1.

J. De Costa et al, 'Women in Surgery: Challenges and opportunities', International Journal of Surgery: Global Health, 2018, vol. 1.

G-R. Joliat et al, 'Systematic Review of the Impact of Patient Death on Surgeons', British Journal of Surgery, 2019, vol. 106, no. 11, pp. 1429–1432.

R. Liang et al, 'Why Do Women Leave Surgical Training? A qualitative and feminist study', The Lancet, 2019, vol. 393, no. 10171, pp. 541–549.

R. Mitchell, 'The Case of the Missing Trainees', presentation to the Royal Australasian College of Surgeons Annual Scientific Congress, 5–9 May 2014.

J. Paik, 'The Feminization of Medicine', *JAMA*, 2000, vol. 283, no. 5, p. 666.

J. Pegrum and O. Pearce, 'A Stressful Job: Are surgeons psychopaths?' The Bulletin of the Royal College of Surgeons of England, vol. 97, no. 8.

C. A. Pfortmueller et al, 'Sexual Activity-related Emergency Department Admissions: Eleven years of experience at a Swiss university hospital', *Emergency Medicine Journal: EMJ*, 2013, vol. 30, no. 10, pp. 846–850.

H. Sarsons, 'Interpreting Signals in the Labor Market: Evidence from medical referrals', Harvard University, working paper, last updated 28 November 2017, accessed 14 February 2022.

C. E. Sharoky et al, 'Does Surgeon Sex Matter?: Practice patterns and outcomes of female and male surgeons', *Annals of Surgery*, 2018, vol. 267, no. 6, pp. 1069–1076.

L. A. Simpson and L. Grant, 'Sources and Magnitude of Job Stress among Physicians', *Journal of Behavioral Medicine*, 1991, vol. 14, no. 1, pp. 27–42.

Y. Tsugawa et al, 'Comparison of Hospital Mortality and Readmission Rates for Medicare Patients Treated by Male vs Female Physicians', *JAMA Intern Med*, 2017, vol. 177, no. 2, pp. 206–213.

C. Wallis et al, 'Comparison of Postoperative Outcomes Among Patients Treated by Male and Female Surgeons: A population based matched cohort study', *The BMJ*, 2017, vol. 359.

C. Wallis et al, 'Association of Surgeon–Patient Sex Concordance with Postoperative Outcomes', *JAMA Surgery*, 2022, vol. 157, no. 2, pp. 146–156.